My Pelvic Flaw

Preventing Pelvic Floor
Problems Throughout Life

by

Mary O'Dwyer
Pelvic Floor Physiotherapist

MY PELVIC FLAW:
PREVENTING PELVIC FLOOR PROBLEMS THROUGHOUT LIFE

First published in 2007
Revised 2008
By Redsok Publishing
PO Box 1881.
Buderim, Queensland, Australia 4556
www.redsok.com.au

National Library of Australia Cataloguing-in-Publication Data

O'Dwyer, Mary Rose.
   My pelvic [floor] flaw: preventing pelvic floor problems throughout life.
   Bibliography.
   1. Pelvic floor - Care and hygiene.
   2. Pelvic floor - Health aspects.
   3. Pelvic floor - Diseases - Prevention.
   4. Pelvic floor - Diseases - Treatment.
   II. Title.   617.55

ISBN 978-0-980399-90-5

Illustrations by Maggie Allingham
Photography by Barry Alsop
Cover Design by Portable Creations
Editing by Word Factory and Gail Tagarro

Disclaimer
All names used in the case studies are fictional. This book represents research and clinical experience, is intended for educational use and is designed to help the reader make informed decisions. This book is not intended as a substitute for treatment by a pelvic floor physiotherapist or doctor.
The publisher, author and distributors expressly disclaim any liability to any person for any injury or inconvenience sustained, or for any use or misuse of any information contained in this book. The author has made every effort to provide accurate and clear information in the book, and cannot be responsible for any misinformation.

This book is a work of non-fiction.
The author asserts her moral rights.

About the author

Mary O'Dwyer, pelvic floor physiotherapist, trained at the Universities of Queensland and Melbourne.

Mary has over 30 years' clinical and teaching experience. Currently consulting in Women's Health at Physiocare, Maroochydore, she is also a Senior Teaching Fellow at Bond University, Gold Coast.

Mary conducts seminars teaching physiotherapists about the pelvic floor and back pain, and fitness professionals about the effects of exercise on the pelvic floor. She also teaches Tai Chi for arthritis, Pilates-based pelvic floor exercise classes and strength training classes for women.

Having witnessed the effect of pelvic floor dysfunction from her patients' stories, Mary is determined to educate women about their pelvic floor health, to enlighten and empower them in the management of relevant problems, while giving them the confidence to make informed decisions.

CONTENTS

8

Introduction

A tight, drawn-in stomach after eight years of classical ballet, three large babies birthed in damaging positions, 10 years of traditional gym work that majored in sit-ups, and restoring an acre of overgrown garden resulted in my own pelvic floor damage.

I realised there must be something missing from my education for this to happen to a fit, healthy physiotherapist.

So I undertook postgraduate study on the pelvic floor and it has changed my focus when treating pelvic floor disorders. Talking to my patients, I learned the extent of pelvic floor dysfunction and the impact that bladder and bowel incontinence, sexual dysfunction and pelvic pain have on women's relationships, self-image and independence. What amazed me was how women poured out their problems, relieved by the opportunity to discuss their issues with someone who wanted to know.

I discovered that women generally accepted pelvic floor problems as part of being female. I learned that vaginal and genital prolapse are waiting to happen in many women, given the 'right' circumstances and especially as they age. We are aware that our mothers and grandmothers experienced prolapse, had hysterectomies or became incontinent as they aged. Secretly, we feared it could become our own destiny as well. But then, we could fix these problems with surgery, couldn't we? However, not all women want to consider this option, as they know someone who has experienced failed surgery, prolapse after hysterectomy, or are unable to have intercourse due to postoperative vaginal pain.

So I asked the question, what could make the difference for us, and for our daughters and granddaughters?

Women need practical knowledge about what causes pelvic floor damage and how to prevent it.

I wrote this book to give women that essential knowledge so they can control their own pelvic floor function throughout their lives and make decisions based on correct information.

I urge you to make this information a part of your female wisdom; talk about it and ensure it is passed on between generations of women.

This information is based on research, studies and clinical findings. Read it one chapter at a time, and practise the steps outlined. Revisit the book often, and re-read the instructions until the message and exercise steps become clear.

My Pelvic Flaw

Most women do not think about their pelvic floor until something goes wrong with it. In fact, they are generally unaware of how this most central part of their body functions.

The problem is not the pelvic floor. The problem is the pelvic FLAW. This flaw is the lack of knowledge; this flaw is faulty movement patterns you have developed throughout life; this flaw is accepting incorrect exercise advice; this flaw is believing your problems can be 'fixed' by surgery while continuing damaging habits.

Your pelvic floor is the centre of your femaleness, so you need the right information to protect it from damage due to exercise, childbirth, menopause and aging. Women are living longer and evidence shows that age increases the risk of developing genital prolapse, resulting in varying symptoms including loss of bladder and bowel control and sexual dysfunction.

Have you thought how life revolves around the pelvic floor? You were supported by, and then delivered through your mother's pelvic floor. At birth, your pelvic floor identified you as female. Significant developmental changes took place at adolescence with the start of your fertility. Exquisite pleasure (unfortunately pain for some) is experienced through your pelvic floor. Your babies are supported by, then birthed through your pelvic floor, and changes again take place at menopause with the cessation of fertility (thank God, I hear you sigh).

Our female pelvic floor dysfunction is often accepted, as we continue to put up with this malfunctioning as part of 'being female'. We are too ashamed to speak with our friends and partners when problems occur. Instead, we put up with ongoing dysfunction for years before seeking help. This book is an attempt to break the cycle of ignorance and give women the knowledge and practical skills to understand and protect their pelvic floor from unnecessary and sometimes self-inflicted damage.

The aim of this book is to provide you with a step-by-step guide to finding, correctly activating and strengthening your pelvic floor muscles and adopting healthy daily habits, as well as practical knowledge to protect your pelvic floor through your life stages. Hopefully, you will apply this knowledge to your own body, teach your daughters and talk to the other women in your life. Maybe then, this knowledge will become part of your everyday lives, female knowledge that is readily discussed among women.

Prolapse, loss of continence, loss of sexual function and the resulting poor quality of life should not be accepted as the consequence of childbirth, over-activity or aging. Your pelvic floor is a part of your body that has special requirements to ensure that it will continue to function with peak efficiency throughout your life.

Are you thinking that *you* won't be affected by pelvic floor dysfunction?

Following childbirth, 50% of women have pelvic organ prolapse, with symptoms of bladder and bowel dysfunction.[1.] In women with vaginal prolapse, 63% will have urinary stress incontinence.[2]

Even though you constantly hear about the importance of doing pelvic floor exercises, the majority of women who visit my clinic just don't know where to find these muscles, or are using the wrong muscles. Research shows that it is difficult and sometimes impossible for women to learn these exercises from a brochure. After giving birth, you are told, 'Don't forget your pelvic floor exercises'. However, if these muscles are cut, swollen and painful, then you might as well have been asked to do brain surgery – you simply don't know how! So, you forget about your pelvic floor and get busy with life, even though you know your pelvic floor does not feel quite the same as it did prior to giving birth.

But surgery can fix it, I hear you say?

Certainly, repair surgery will help many women regain their control and dignity, but it is also fraught with problems. In addition, an estimated 30% of operations fail and are repeated.[3] Why not learn the everyday steps to help control symptoms before they require surgery?

Take responsibility for your pelvic floor today and continue the daily habits you are about to learn for the rest of your life. The easy-to-follow, step-by-step programme outlined in the following chapters will give you the important facts and strategies to help prevent, and maybe overcome your own pelvic floor dysfunction.

Women who have been subject to sexual abuse can experience higher rates of pelvic pain, overactive bladder, bowel dysfunction and hypertonic (too tight) pelvic floor muscles. Hypertonic muscles initially require relaxation before learning the correct pattern of contraction. If you suffer from undiagnosed pelvic pain, bladder urgency and leaking, I encourage you to consult a gynaecologist and pelvic floor physiotherapist for specific treatment (refer to the section on *Pain and the Pelvic Floor*, page 89).

This book is intended as an adjunct to, and not a replacement for consultation with a pelvic floor physiotherapist or gynaecologist. The contents of the book are based on the findings of researchers and my own clinical knowledge.

My thanks go to clients and friends for urging me to write this book, to my dear husband for his constant support and to the multitude of researchers, whose findings underpin my clinical work.

My dream is that the information you are about to read becomes common knowledge amongst women. Congratulations on buying this book. Please put the information into practice and recommend it to the women in your life. Talk to your mothers, daughters, friends, cousins and aunts. I thank you for helping this information become part of our female wisdom.

What is the Pelvic Floor?

The pelvic floor is the platform of muscles and sphincters of your bladder and urethra, vagina and anus. It involves the network of muscles, ligaments and fascia (fascia is the tough, thin, translucent membrane similar to what you pull off meat) that supports your bladder, vagina, uterus and bowel.

The pelvic floor is one group of muscles that is rarely trained. Many women have no idea of pelvic floor tensioning before activity and during exercise. Due to poor posture, straining to open the bowel, incorrect breathing patterns and inappropriate exercise, they learn to substitute stronger outer tummy muscles for the correct pelvic floor action. This substitution occurs if the waist is constantly drawn back in an attempt to make the tummy look flatter.

Researchers are now identifying a high rate of pelvic floor dysfunction in these women.[4]

If you have delivered even one baby with tearing, stitches or instrumental delivery, then you have a higher risk of developing pelvic floor problems.[5]

Excess weight, prolonged coughing, repeated heavy lifting, constipation, muscle weakness, connective tissue weakness or previous pelvic surgery can all contribute to pelvic floor dysfunction.

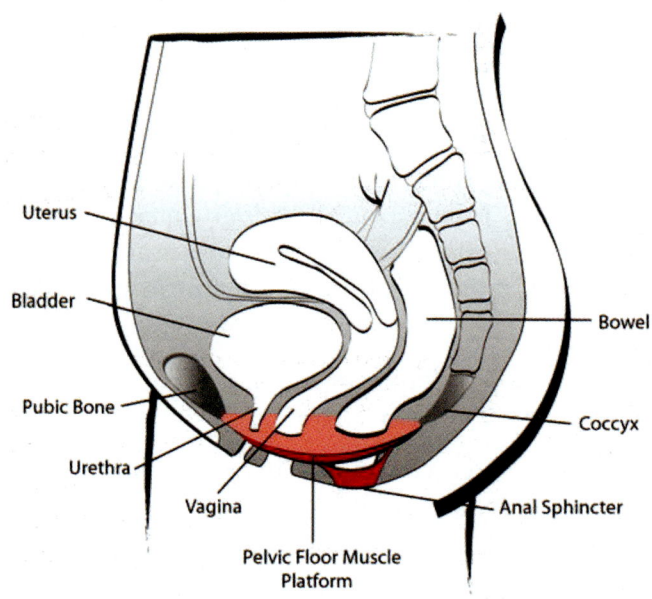

Uterus

Bladder

Pubic Bone

Urethra

Vagina

Pelvic Floor Muscle
Platform

Bowel

Coccyx

Anal Sphincter

Fig. 1 - Pelvic Floor, side view

What is Pelvic Floor Dysfunction?

It is any urinary or faecal incontinence or obstruction, constipation, vaginal or uterine prolapse, vaginal or rectal pain, sexual dysfunction or pelvic pain.

Pelvic floor dysfunction can present in children and teenagers, in athletes, during pregnancy or after birth. It may present or worsen during the menopausal years, or become evident after abdominal or pelvic surgery, spinal injury and prolonged bed rest or with aging.

Incorrect toileting habits learned in childhood, inappropriate exercise, habitual slumping and prolonged coughing, repeated heavy lifting, and inheriting poor collagen all contribute to pelvic floor dysfunction.

So What Goes Wrong?

Weakness

Some women may have developed weak pelvic floor muscles in childhood, caused by straining to empty their bowel, as a result of slumped posture or chronic coughing. Some might inherit weaker collagen, increasing the risk of dysfunction. Because the pelvic floor is one of the most forgotten muscle groups in the body, it wastes away, becoming thinner and weaker.

Ongoing coughing with chest disease (asthma) or a prolonged chest infection causes repeated downward pressure on your pelvic floor. If your pelvic floor is weak, then this downward pressure will further weaken pelvic floor supports. Smokers are more at risk of pelvic floor problems because of repeated coughing. Slumping switches off the pelvic floor and deep abdominal muscles, leading to weakness.[6]

Damage

Regular straining to open the bowel has been shown to progressively damage the nerves that supply pelvic floor muscles. This can cause a loss of bowel control.[7] Straining will also aggravate a bladder prolapse, causing a bulge at the vaginal entrance.

Fat

Excessive abdominal fat creates constant downward pressure on your pelvic floor. Women with a larger waist measurement have a higher risk of pelvic floor dysfunction. Overweight women often show a significant improvement of continence when they lose weight.

Lifting

Heavy lifting causes a strong internal downward pressure on the pelvic floor. Women can have weaker pelvic muscles and tears in supporting fascia after childbirth. Continuing to lift heavy weights causes more strain and damage to a pre-weakened pelvic floor.

Childbirth

Damage may occur with childbirth. Fascia and muscle can be strained during pregnancy, or torn, cut and stitched at the time of delivery. Nerves can be damaged by stretching or cutting, so that the pelvic floor muscles are much weaker and don't always automatically start working again.

Why is Pelvic Floor Dysfunction a Problem?

While pelvic floor dysfunction may be no more than a nuisance to some women, others find that it can increasingly affect their quality of life.

- It might limit their choice of sport or activity, leading to weight gain.

- Due to loss of confidence, some women do not venture far from home and pass up opportunities to travel.

- Frequent toilet visits at night will cause disturbed sleep patterns and ongoing fatigue.

- Relationships can suffer through loss of intimacy, leading to anxiety and personality changes.

- Chronic pelvic pain can cause depression and negative thinking.

- The added expense of buying continence products will be a burden to women on a limited income.

There is no one particular treatment for all pelvic floor problems. If a woman has a weak pelvic floor, she will benefit from strength training. However, another woman may have a tight, painful pelvic floor due to constant muscle tension. Strength training would make her worse. Another woman might substitute other muscles for the pelvic floor, and will need to learn to locate and coordinate the pelvic floor with other core muscles first, before she strengthens.

Correct identification of any dysfunction first, is critical to ensure the correct therapy.

The Role of your Pelvic Floor

1. The pelvic floor is the muscular platform that supports your bladder, vagina, uterus and bowel. When you tension your pelvic floor muscles, this tensioning should close the sphincters of these organs and maintain your continence.

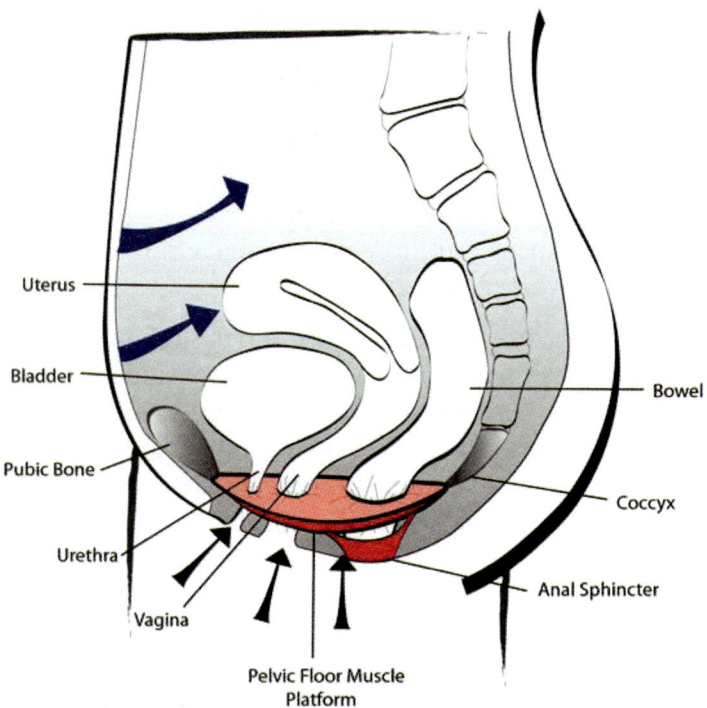

The Pelvic Floor Muscle Platform contracts to close the urethral and anal sphincters and draw up the vaginal walls.

Fig. 2 - Pelvic Floor Elevation

2. It tensions with your deep abdominal muscle (Transversus abdominis), your diaphragm and deep spinal muscles to form an internal cylinder that supports your spine.[8]

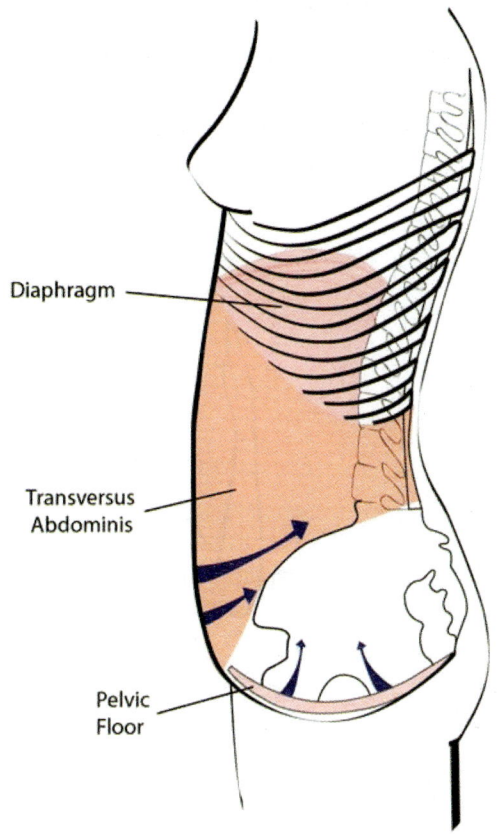

Diaphragm

Transversus
Abdominis

Pelvic
Floor

The action of Pelvic Floor and Transversus is to tension
up and brace against downward internal pressure.

Fig. 3 - Inner Cylinder of 'Core' Muscles

3. It resists downward internal pressure on your pelvic organs when you cough, lift or run.

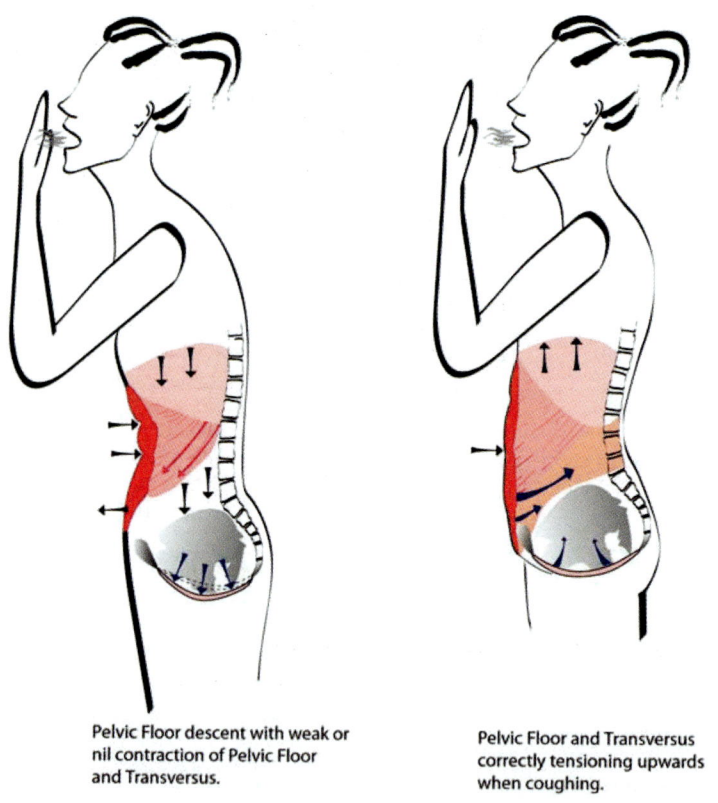

Pelvic Floor descent with weak or nil contraction of Pelvic Floor and Transversus.

Pelvic Floor and Transversus correctly tensioning upwards when coughing.

Fig. 4 – Incorrect and Correct Muscle Action with Coughing

4. The muscles direct blood flow to your clitoris and contract to give you orgasmic sensations.

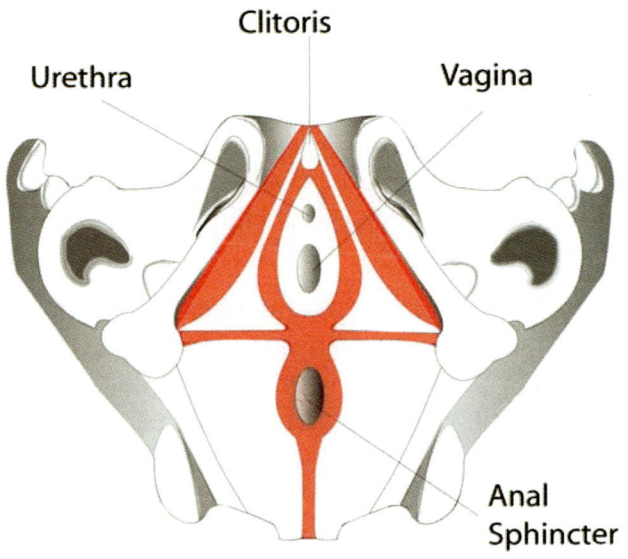

Outer layer of muscles that direct
blood flow to the clitoris

Fig. 5 - Pelvic Floor, viewed from below

23

Horrible Pelvic Floor Habits

1. *Regularly stopping your urine flow* to exercise your pelvic floor muscles is not a healthy habit. Your urine should empty freely as your bladder contracts. Only OCCASIONALLY use 'stopping your flow' as a test to gauge your level of control. When passing urine, never push down to empty your bladder, just relax your abdomen forwards.

2. *Hovering over the toilet.* Some women avoid sitting on a public toilet seat, however hovering above the seat makes it difficult for your bladder to empty. The best option is to take your own disposable toilet seat liners, so you can sit and relax to empty your bladder effectively. To empty your bladder fully, sit upright with your sternum lifted and completely relax your waist and abdomen. Your bladder will then contract to empty the urine. A slower urine stream can be due to prolapse and weak pelvic floor muscles.

3. *'I do my pelvic floor exercises while I'm driving or at the traffic lights'.* I don't advise this, as the car seat typically puts you in the slump position and this lets your outer tummy muscles take over the exercise. If you only ever do your exercises in the car, then you will never learn to strengthen in standing. Initially many women need to learn the correct tensioning pattern sitting or lying on their side. After you learn this correct tensioning, start the tensioning in standing. Why? Because your pelvic floor has to do most work in standing, moving, lifting and bending. In standing, your pelvic floor has greater demands placed on it to tension and firmly hold up against the downwards intra-abdominal pressure. Make time to

give the exercises your total focus and keep repeating them daily while standing.

4. *Slumping in sitting.* This shuts down your core, supporting muscles. It's up to you now to regain control over your lower back and spine, by retraining yourself to sit and stand upright. (It also helps you feel more confident – try it). Be smarter in the chairs you choose to support your spine. Best choice is a straight-backed chair with support up to, but below, your shoulder blades. Lounge chairs with a high headrest push your spine into a slumped or 'C' curved position. Keep both feet flat on the floor. Only cross your legs for short periods if you can maintain an upright spinal position. When your back tires, place a support or pillow in your low back and still keep your sternum lifted. Remember to relax your waist in sitting, and let your deep abdominal and pelvic floor muscles provide the correct spinal support.

Many women do not realise they hold constant tension at their waist and the base of their ribs. This incorrect tension will change the normal diaphragmatic breathing pattern and in time change the coordination of your diaphragm, pelvic floor and deep abdominal muscles. Constant waist tension recruits the wrong muscles and alters the coordination of your inner and outer abdominal muscles.

5. *Curl-ups.* Forget curl-ups, crunches or sit-ups for abdominal strengthening. The women who focus on crunches, incline bench sit-ups, medicine ball curls or double leg lifts, typically struggle to learn pelvic floor tensioning. These exercises are damaging for many women and repeatedly force strong pressure down on to your pelvic floor. Stop straining already weakened tissues. Making the outer trunk muscles super strong can lead to a muscle imbalance problem. Your focus needs to be on the

deep abdominal (and pelvic floor) as this is the muscle that flattens your tummy. Crunches will not shift abdominal fat.

Important Tip

When doing any exercise, be aware of whether your pelvic floor holds or if it pushes down. If it pushes down, then that exercise is too difficult for your pelvic floor, and you need a more suitable activity.

6. *A tight waist.* A constantly drawn in, tight waist is perhaps women's WORST habit. Why? Researchers have observed women with pelvic floor problems habitually use their outer abdominal muscles to tighten or draw in their waist when they perform any forceful action such as lifting, carrying, pushing or coughing. This forces pressure down internally, overwhelming the pelvic floor. Women without pelvic floor problems however, automatically use their pelvic floor and inner abdominal muscles when they lift or cough[76].

Think of your abdomen as a balloon. The top of the balloon is your domed diaphragm, the round part is your deep abdominal muscle and the under part of the balloon is your pelvic floor. Place the balloon beneath a ledge or shelf so the top is up against the barrier. Now place your hands around the 'waist' of the balloon and slowly squeeze in. Notice how the under part bulges down. This is the effect on your pelvic floor of tightening the waist. Learning to consciously release and soften your waist is perhaps the most difficult habit of all to change as your brain has learned to pull the waist back on exertion. Take a moment to look at a child's relaxed waist then look in the mirror to see the difference at your waist.

26

The Steps to Learning the Correct Pelvic Floor Action

To do these steps, sit in front of a mirror so that you can observe what happens in your abdomen.

1. Posture

Learn to keep your inner postural muscles switched on by continuing to control your upright spinal posture in sitting, then in standing.

Keep your body weight down through the sitting bones under your butt, not slumped and rolled back onto your sacrum. Slumping shuts down your inner postural muscles and lets your pelvic floor sag.

After you tilt your pelvis forwards over the sitting bones, lift up your sternum and hold as you release your waist and soften your abdomen forwards. This is important to break the hold of your outer tummy muscles. Are you really uncomfortable about letting your tummy go soft? O.K. You have been told all your life to pull your stomach in, but you have learned to overuse the outer abdominal instead of being taught to tension the inner abdominal. Let go of the outer waist tightness. Switch off this hyperactive muscle in order to feel the gentler inner abdominal tensioning (Transversus abdominis), because this is the muscle that correctly flattens your tummy.

As seen in Fig. 6, sitting upright switches on your deep abdominal and pelvic floor muscles. Sitting and standing tall are the correct endurance exercises for these deep muscles.

27

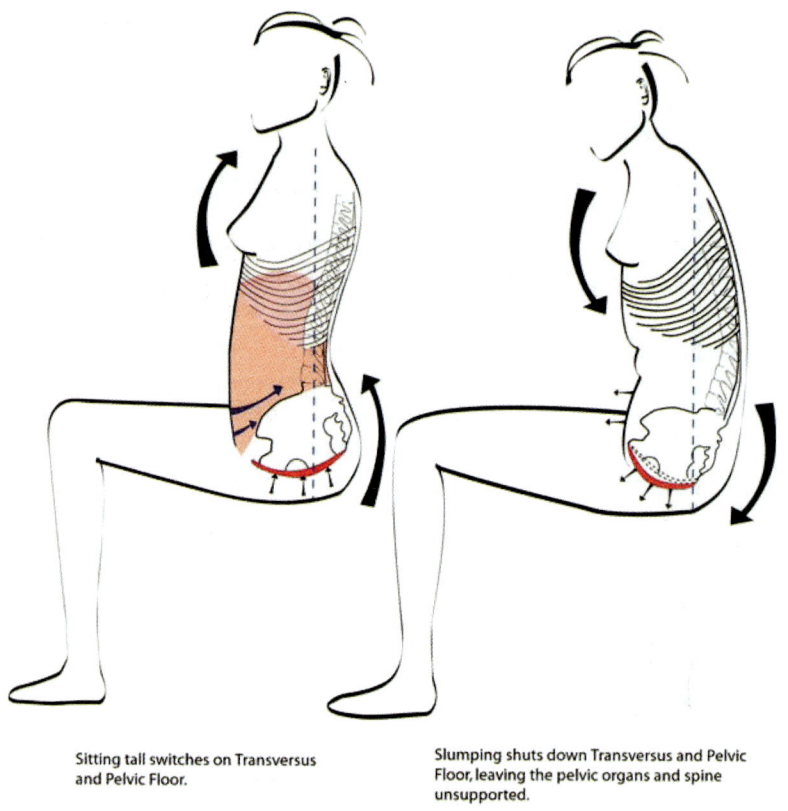

Sitting tall switches on Transversus and Pelvic Floor.

Slumping shuts down Transversus and Pelvic Floor, leaving the pelvic organs and spine unsupported.

Fig. 6 - Sitting Posture and the Pelvic Floor

2. Correct breathing

When you breathe, the base of your ribs and abdomen should open up as your shoulders stay relaxed. If you constantly pull your stomach in at the waist, then you probably lift up your chest and shoulders when you breathe in.

This incorrect pattern of breathing stops your diaphragm from smoothly moving up and down.

Correct Breathing Pattern   Incorrect Breathing Pattern

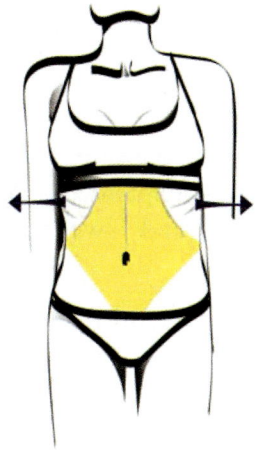
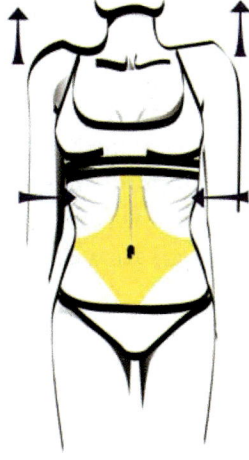

Ribs open out sideways   Waist draws in, rib cage and
and stomach swells.   shoulders lift up.

Fig. 7 - Breathing Patterns

Guess what?

Your diaphragm and pelvic floor move together. If your diaphragm is not free to move DOWN when you breathe in, and UP under your lungs when you breathe out, you will not be able to effectively tension your pelvic floor. The diaphragm does not move correctly if you lift up your chest and shoulders while tightening in at your waist. Your diaphragm moves correctly when you expand and open up your abdomen and the base of your ribs as you breathe in.

If you are a chronic slumper, then your diaphragm has no room to move down when you breathe in. This in turn prevents your pelvic floor muscles from working correctly. By now, you're probably hearing your mother's constant reminders about sitting up straight.

To learn the correct pattern of opening up the base of your ribs when breathing in, start by watching your chest and ribs in the mirror. If your chest and shoulders lift when you breathe in, you have an incorrect pattern of breathing.

Sit and place a tape measure around the base of your ribs. When you breathe in slowly and deeply, expand the tape by opening your lower ribs to the side and swelling your abdominal wall forwards (see Fig. 8).

Continue to repeat and learn this breathing until it becomes your regular pattern. Initially this can be difficult if your breathing muscles are tight and/or weak. Do you get breathless when you exercise? This might be due to your tight upper-chest breathing pattern preventing you from taking an effective deep breath.

If you are unable to learn a smooth, easy pattern of breathing in sitting, lie down on your back with both knees bent. Place your hands on your abdomen, over the base of your ribs. Observe what happens under your hands. Start to gently open your ribs and stomach under your hands as you breathe in, and relax slowly as you breathe out. Notice how your pelvic floor gently draws upwards as you breathe out.

When breathing correctly, your outer tummy muscles should release and open as you breathe in, then the inner abdominal and pelvic floor muscles should tension as you breathe out.

Practise the same slow abdominal basal rib breathing in sitting and in standing. When you walk, release any tight waist tension and practice this pattern of breathing.

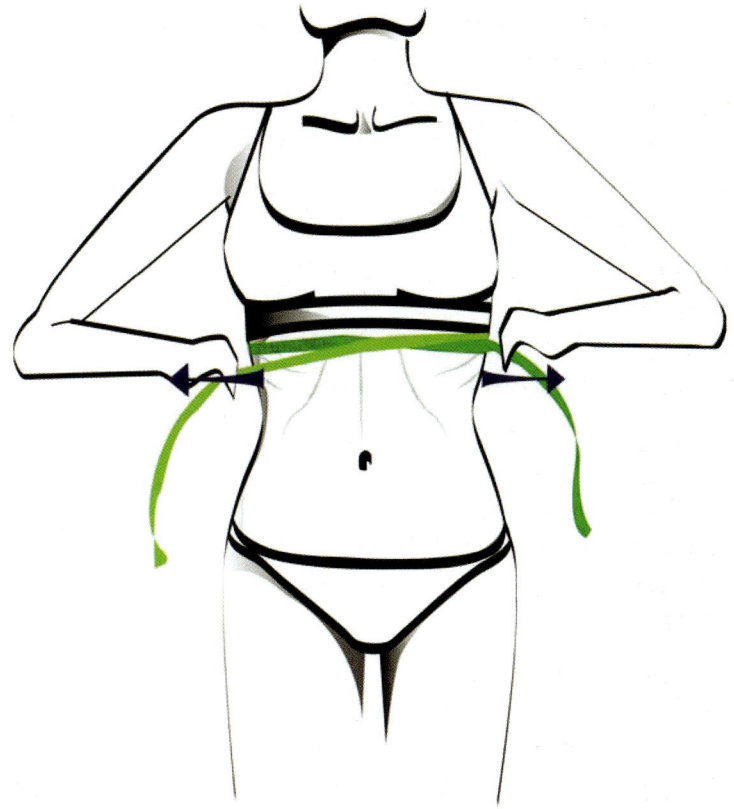

Lower ribs open out on the in breath to expand the tape.
Shoulders stay flat.

Fig. 8 - Learning Correct Breathing

3. Correct Tensioning

Find your pubic bone, then move in under the bone and gently push up on the end of your urethra (this is where your urine exits). It is located behind your clitoris and in front of your vaginal opening. Now take your other hand and find your coccyx at the base or your spine (this is up behind your anal sphincter).

When you start to gently tension your pelvic floor muscles, this is where you will start to slowly tension FIRST. As you breathe out, gently draw your pubic bone back towards your coccyx. (Remember this is slow and gentle in this learning stage, because you need to learn what these muscles feel like without the bullying waist muscles jumping in to take over).

If you are tensioning correctly, you will feel your lower abdominal wall gently tension back (above your pubic bone). If you try too hard or too fast, your waist will take over the task.

If you find it's difficult to locate your gentle pelvic floor muscles with this tensioning, then imagine a sharp needle coming towards your urethra. Slowly draw your urethra away from the needle as you breathe out.

Substitution

So what happens when these muscles are too weak or uncoordinated to work effectively? Outer abdominal muscles will take over the role and you learn (incorrectly) to use these strong outer muscles instead of the gentle inner abdominal and pelvic floor muscles. Look at your child's stomach and observe their rounded tummy. Notice how the waist is relaxed, as children have not learned the incorrect waist tension used by so many adults in a misguided attempt to flatten their stomachs.

Fig. 9 shows the incorrect outer tummy muscle substitution. This substitution becomes automatic with lifting and coughing, causing a lifetime pattern of internal pressure down on the pelvic floor. If the pelvic floor is unable to tension upwards to counteract this pressure, the pelvic organs cannot be effectively supported. Likewise, the lumbar spine and sacro-iliac joints need the same deep abdominal and pelvic floor tensioning to stabilise and protect the spine during movement.

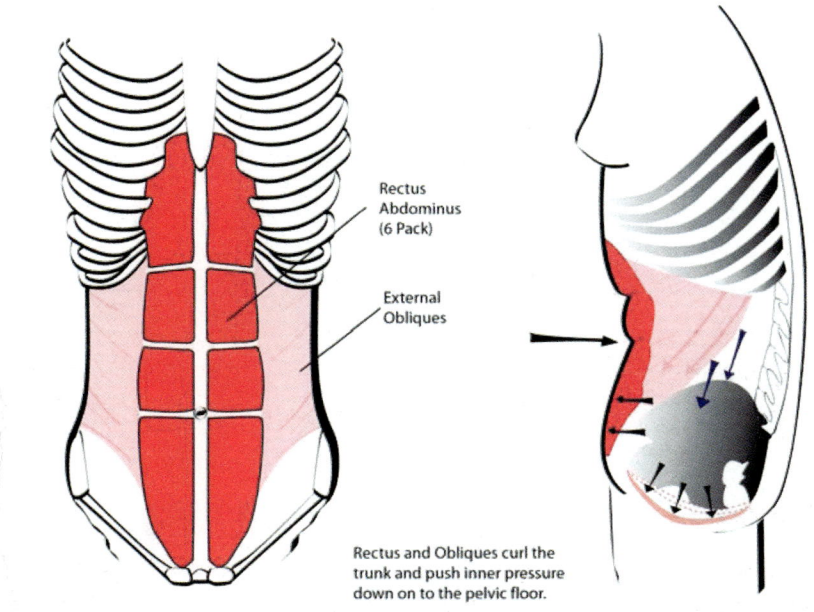

Rectus
Abdominus
(6 Pack)

External
Obliques

Rectus and Obliques curl the
trunk and push inner pressure
down on to the pelvic floor.

Fig. 9 - Outer Abdominal Muscles used in Waist Tensioning

The next diagram shows the tensioning that should occur between the pelvic floor and deep abdominal muscle. Every woman should learn this tensioning to use before coughing, pushing, lifting and sneezing.

This tensioning should happen before you lift a weight at the gym, as you dig in the garden, as you pick up a toddler or turn the mattress on your bed.

Using this correct muscle pattern will protect your back when you lift as well as keeping you continent when sneezing.

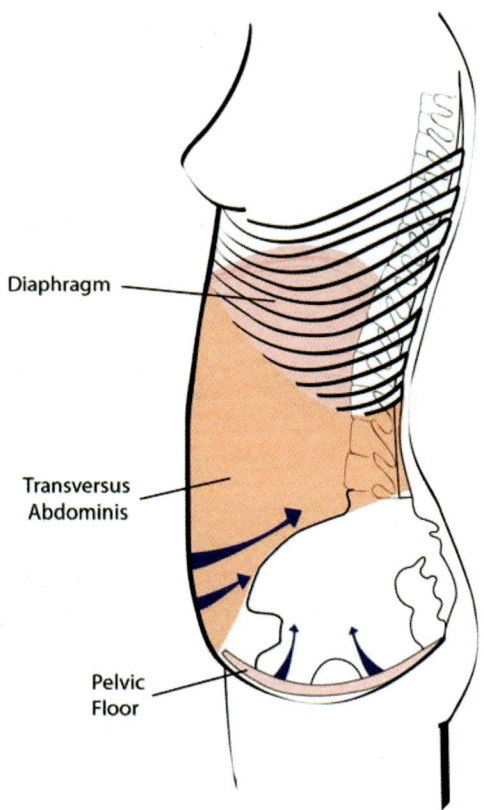

Diaphragm

Transversus
Abdominis

Pelvic
Floor

The action of Pelvic Floor and Transversus is to tension
up and brace against downward internal pressure.

Fig. 10 - Inner Cylinder Core Muscles

Why is substitution a problem?

Continuing to use and tighten the outer abdominals (when your
pelvic floor is weak or uncoordinated) will force pressure
downwards onto your pelvic floor. So, when you lift a heavy

object or cough strongly, the outer abdominal muscles contract strongly, without the stabilising effect of the inner pelvic and deep abdominal muscles. Over time, this will stretch the ligaments that support your pelvic organs from above. If these ligaments are stretched, they cannot support your bladder, vagina, uterus and bowel, leaving you more prone to prolapse.

Researchers have analysed which muscles incontinent women use to tension their pelvic floor[9] and found that:

- Four out of 10 women tighten their outer tummy and chest wall muscles and incorrectly bear down on their pelvic floor.

- Two out of 10 women have no contraction in their pelvic floor.

- Four out of 10 women have the correct action of tensioning up their pelvic floor and deep abdominal muscle.

So,

Six out of 10 women need to learn how to retrain the normal pattern of tensioning for their internal muscles.

Why is this so difficult?

It is difficult because it involves learning to use different muscles from the ones that your body and brain now **automatically** use to tension your pelvic floor.

Women who have learned a pattern of using outer tummy muscles to bear down (instead of tensioning upwards) will have the most difficulty learning the correct pattern. Be patient when learning and don't give up. You will notice an improvement in your problematic bladder and bowel when you learn to use your pelvic floor muscles correctly.

Many women try far too hard when learning pelvic floor exercises and end up tightening waist, leg and buttock muscles. This only reinforces the incorrect pattern of bearing down.

Important Tip

> **Your inner cylinder muscles don't tighten hard and fast like the muscles that move you. These inner (postural) muscles tension SLOWLY AND GENTLY.**

So, you must forget about strength in the early LEARNING stage. You will never find these inner muscles if you use any more than a very slow, gentle drawing action. This stage of learning has nothing to do with strength, rather it is about locating and coordinating the muscles in a gentle manner, so your brain can learn the correct sensation without the stronger outer abdominals taking over.

Don't even try to strengthen until you can find these muscles without the strong outer muscles jumping in first. Only when you can confidently tension the correct muscles, should you start to internally draw and lift these muscles more firmly.

After you learn to correctly tension, the next stage is about improving STRENGTH. Expect that it will take you five to six months of daily maximal lifts to strengthen your pelvic floor significantly.

Strength is gained by correctly using stretch bands, a Pilates ring and fitball. If you have a strongly entrenched pattern of substitution, introducing strength work early will only reinforce the outer abdominal muscle pattern.

Avoid rushing this early learning stage because you cannot progress until you learn the correct tensioning pattern.

Putting it All Together

- Sit upright and keep your sternum lifted as you relax your abdomen forwards.

- You can also start this lying on your side, if sitting does not work for you.

- Breathe in slowly and deeply, expanding the base of your ribs and opening up your abdomen.

- As you breathe out slowly, leave your waist soft and slowly draw your pubic bone back towards your coccyx, to feel how your vagina and urethra tension and draw slightly in an upwards direction.

You may respond better to different cues. Imagine a sharp needle coming towards your urethra and slowly drawing away from it. Or imagine a line connecting your front hip bones; as you breathe out, slowly shorten this line as if to draw your hip bones closer together. Learn to hold this tension as you breathe.

If performed correctly, you will feel a gentle urethral and vaginal lifting and tensioning above your pubic bone in the lower abdomen. This is Transversus Abdominis tensioning with your pelvic floor.[10] If you try this too fast or too hard, then your waist muscles will jump in to perform the task.

Relax and start again until you can feel the gentle tension between your pelvic floor and deep tummy muscle. Many of my clients say, 'But I hardly feel anything', to which I always reply, 'That's it'. This is a slow, very gentle tensioning in this early learning stage. The sensation is totally different from what you feel when you tighten a strength muscle.

Hold this light tension as you return to rib opening breathing.

Hold for 10 seconds as you breathe, repeat five times and do the exercise three or four times during your day.

Important Tip

If your muscles let go when you breathe, you are probably using the outer tummy muscles instead of the gentler inner ones. Stop, and start again.

Start by lying on your side and then try it in a sitting position for at least a few weeks before practising this same tensioning in standing.

Many women can correctly tension their pelvic floor in sitting. However, when they stand up, this puts more pressure downwards onto the floor, so they incorrectly substitute the waist muscles again.

So expect to find pelvic floor tensioning more difficult when standing, as your strong outer tummy muscles are programmed to take over the task. If you find the tensioning is easier to do while standing then you are probably doing it incorrectly.

Remember to use the mirror to see if the waist muscles draw in first to do the task. Be patient, and tension slowly and gently from the urethra first.

These exercises will force you to stop, slow down and recognise the tension that you unknowingly hold around your waist and ribs. Most of the female population tries to flatten their tummy by pulling their waist back strongly. This is the wrong place to tension – let your waist relax and use pelvic floor and deep abdominal tension instead. Remember to practise upright sitting because this position lets your pelvic floor muscles work more effectively. A slumped posture shuts these muscles down.[6] You have more chance of success with these exercises if you relax and breathe correctly first.

Avoid wearing a tight bra or tight belts around your waist and ribs, as this prevents your lower ribs from opening up when you breathe in.

BE PATIENT with yourself in this learning stage. Let go of frustration, as it takes time to re-programme your brain to recognise these gentle muscles and learn a different action. Initially your brain may not know what you are trying to do, as it does not recognise the location or gentle drawing action of these muscles.

Close your eyes, then go back to relaxing your waist and slower basal rib breathing before trying again.

Remember, your pelvic floor muscles do not work alone. To be effective you must learn to coordinate their action with your diaphragm, abdominal, chest wall and deep spinal muscles. (This is where correct posture and breathing help). If this does not happen after you practise all the earlier steps, then it is time to consult a pelvic floor physiotherapist.

Ten Healthy Habits
for the Pelvic Floor

1. Change your Toilet Position

Before Thomas Crapper introduced the toilet to nineteenth-century London, people would squat to empty their bowel. Squatting puts your bowel in the right position to empty more easily and completely.

If your habit is to slump and strain to empty your bowel, then you risk aggravating bladder incontinence, rectal and/or vaginal prolapse.

Start adopting this new position every day to empty your bowel.

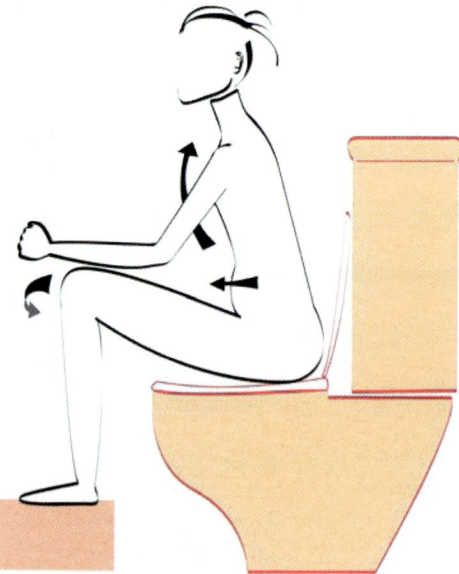

Fig. 11 - Correct Toilet Position

- Place your feet on a stool

- Straighten your lower back and lift up your sternum

- Now open your knees wide, and lean forward from your hips (keep your sternum up)

- Breathe deeply – open abdomen and base of ribs – and totally relax your abdomen forwards.

Avoid slumping your lower back or drawing your waist backwards, as this will close the anal sphincter. You need a relaxed, open sphincter for efficient bowel emptying.[11]

Your bowel will not empty just because you decide that it should. Give yourself time; don't force the issue. Some mothers let their demanding toddlers sit on their knee at the same time, or rush toileting because of a busy schedule. This only causes abdominal tension, which makes bowel emptying more difficult and promotes straining.

When washing your hands after toileting, tension your anal sphincter and slowly draw up through your back passage. Hold and breathe for 10 seconds, every time after your bowel empties.

If you have a slower emptying bowel, then you need to look at:

- increasing your fibre levels

- increasing your water intake

- starting regular exercise; and

- adopting the new toilet position with waist relaxation.

For more information about CONSTIPATION, go to:

www.aboutconstipation.org/characteristics.html

After childbirth and pelvic repair surgery, or if you have a vaginal prolapse, protect your pelvic floor when your bowel opens. Wrap toilet paper around your hand and firmly support your vaginal area while your bowel opens.

If your bowel matter is soft and still does not empty, then you may have a back vaginal wall prolapse that requires pressure on your back vaginal wall to assist emptying.

Ongoing constipation and emptying problems require review by a gynaecologist and pelvic floor physiotherapist.

□ **Case Study** □

Eileen, a 29-year-old bank manager, was referred by her gastroenterologist for advice about her constipation. She had strained to empty her bowel since childhood. The constant straining had caused her bowel to prolapse forwards into the back of her vaginal wall. She had no children. Examination of her food and fluid diary showed that she ate around 15 grams of fibre daily (we require 30-35 grams daily for a soft bowel motion) and drank only one glass of water daily (mostly drank coffee or soft drink). She worked long hours and gave no priority to her need for regular exercise.

To empty her bowel she slumped, strongly pulled her waist back and strained down firmly onto a closed anal sphincter. This was the pattern she had used since childhood, as no one had ever shown her how to sit upright and push her tummy forwards.

Eileen began a new routine of six glasses of water daily, ate fruit or vegetables at every meal, and added whole grains and a daily fibre supplement to her diet. She started a walking programme, correct pelvic floor exercises and adopted (for life) the correct position and abdominal relaxation for easier bowel emptying.

At her third visit, Eileen was delighted to report that her bowel was opening without straining, every second day, instead of once every six days.

2. Stop Lifting Heavy Weights

After giving birth vaginally, you no longer have an intact pelvic floor. Every woman who delivers vaginally has some degree of vaginal prolapse. Think of the tough, thin translucent membrane that you pull off meat. (My apologies to all the vegetarian readers.) That is the fascia. It is stretched during pregnancy and can tear as the baby's head is delivered vaginally. (This is what tears when your outer tummy muscles separate during pregnancy). Fascial tears don't repair, so your vaginal walls sag. Whether this progresses onto a more significant prolapse depends on several things: the muscular strength in your pelvic floor; your decision to avoid heavy weights and to stop straining the bowel; controlling your weight gain; and avoiding inappropriate abdominal exercises.

You will need to be vigilant in the months following childbirth. Your pelvic floor muscles may not be activating when you lift toddlers, baby capsules and prams. This is a life stage when you are more at risk of prolapse. Make the decision to AVOID lifting anything heavier than your baby, until you have found and rehabilitated your pelvic floor muscles. Make the decision to stop heavy lifting throughout your life.

Why?

Because lifting heavy weights, like prolonged coughing, straining the bowel and sit-ups all cause heavy pressure down on your pelvic floor from inside your body. I will keep on repeating this message, in the hope that it will imprint strongly in your memory.

Fig. 12 shows how intra abdominal pressure pushes down on the pelvic floor, promoting more damage in the woman who is unable to tension her pelvic floor up against this pressure. This muscle pattern is commonly seen in women with pelvic floor dysfunction. Women without any problems predominantly use their pelvic floor and deep abdominal muscles when they lift or cough.

43

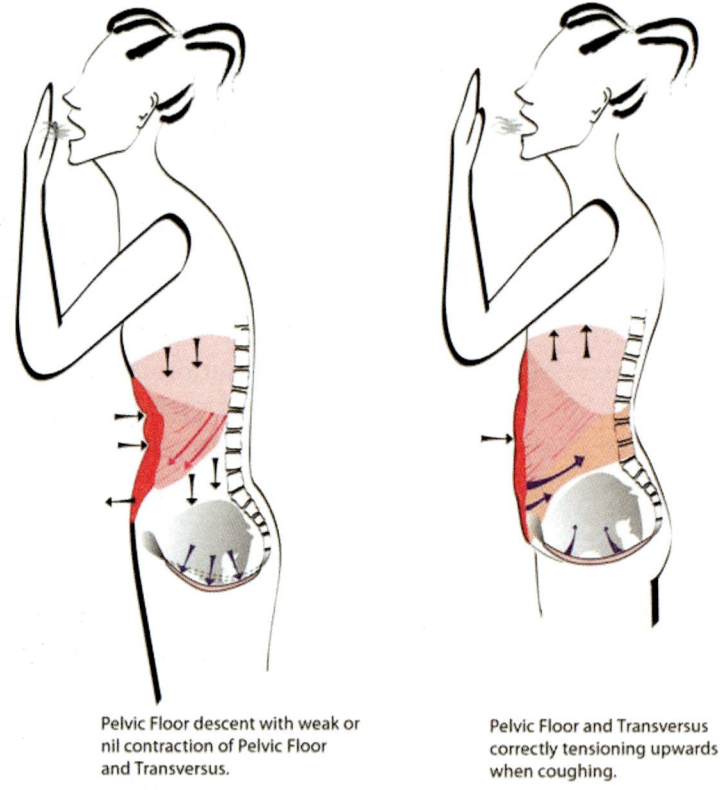

Pelvic Floor descent with weak or
nil contraction of Pelvic Floor
and Transversus.

Pelvic Floor and Transversus
correctly tensioning upwards
when coughing.

Fig. 12 – Coughing and Lifting Muscle Action

A study of assistant nurses in Denmark showed a 60% increased
risk of pelvic organ prolapse and herniated lumbar discs due to
the ongoing heavy lifting at work.[12] Women who work as
labourers and factory workers have a high risk of developing
genital prolapse because of the heavy work and prolonged
standing.[13]

□ Case Study □

Tina was referred three weeks after the birth of her first baby. She
described a wonderful birth, initially in standing, then in a bath,
followed by delivery on all fours. She had bowel pain from an

internal haemorrhoid and was constipated for five days after the birth. A week after returning home, she continued to strain hard to empty her bowel, causing her cervix and uterus to prolapse down into her vagina. Towards the end of each day, she was in pain from the prolapse.

Tina's depressed mood was evident in her slumped sitting posture. To tension her pelvic floor muscles, she used strong outer tummy muscles to pull her waist back. This incorrect muscle substitution pushed her prolapse down further.

Her programme started with controlling her spinal posture in sitting and standing. She stopped lifting any more than her baby, increased her intake of fresh fruit and vegetables, water and fibre, adopted the new toilet position (with hand pressure up over her vagina as her bowel opened) and started correct pelvic floor exercises.

Tina progressed to pelvic floor strength exercises in sitting and standing, and learned to tension her pelvic floor before lifting anything.

She soon reported less pain, and her bowel opened regularly without straining. After months of progressive strength exercises, she was able to lift her heavy baby in his car capsule while holding her pelvic floor tensioned. She started bike riding, walking and swimming for fitness and weight loss. When time allowed she did Fitball and Pilates classes for ongoing strengthening.

Tina and her partner wanted to have a second baby. She decided to wait for 18 months and fully rehabilitate her pelvic floor strength, so that she would be strong enough to carry another baby, knowing she would have to pick up a heavy toddler as well.

3. Never Lift more than your Pelvic Floor can Control

When you lift heavy weights, the pressure that develops inside your abdomen pushes down on your pelvic floor. Without effective pelvic floor muscles to counter that pressure, you risk uterine and/or vaginal prolapse. If your vaginal walls or cervix bulge out of your vaginal entrance, or your rectum protrudes externally, then you have a significant prolapse that may require surgery. You will not always know that you have a prolapse. If you experience urine loss, rectal and/or vaginal pain and heaviness, constipation, discomfort or pain during intercourse, then you may have vaginal prolapse.

In an Australian study, 69% of the women with significant uterine prolapse had a retroverted uterus.[14] The retroverted uterus tips backwards towards the spine (instead of forwards above the bladder). If you are one of the 20%-25% of women who have a retroverted uterus, it is even more important to focus on avoiding the causes of prolapse (page 99) and to commit yourself to a lifetime of pelvic floor exercises.

Think carefully before surgery

Your surgeon may do brilliant repair work, but if you continue to lift heavy weights or strain the bowel with a weak pelvic floor, yes, you guessed it, you are at risk of further prolapse. If you have learned to substitute outer tummy muscles (instead of the correct pelvic floor action), you would be pushing down on the repair instead of supporting the repair.

Not all cases of prolapse require surgery. Some women are able to reduce and maintain the prolapse without surgery, by strengthening their pelvic floor and avoiding aggravating factors.

Women who begin a gym strength programme with a weak pelvic floor, or no knowledge of how to tension and hold these muscles, risk aggravating a pre-existing prolapse. Remember – most women who deliver vaginally have some degree of vaginal prolapse.

If you decide to start gym training, you must train your pelvic floor and deep abdominal muscles FIRST, so you have a protective muscular inner support system when you exercise. Most trainers today are young men and women, with great exercise prescription skills but little knowledge of pelvic floor muscles and the dysfunction caused by inappropriate exercises. Incontinence is considered a taboo topic with many younger, fit people. They are usually too embarrassed to ask relevant questions about your pelvic floor function in the initial assessment prior to exercising.

Important Tip

> **To avoid aggravating prolapse, gym trainers need to ask a series of RED FLAG questions as part of a client's initial assessment.**

RED FLAG questions are ones that alert the trainer to the presence of pelvic floor problems. See these questions in the Gym and Pelvic Floor section (page 91).

Some women who develop prolapse after starting an exercise programme are too embarrassed to mention their vaginal bulge, so they avoid some exercises or decide to stop exercising. Others develop bladder urgency, then urine loss, but do not associate this with their gym work.

If you are told to 'turn on your inner core', by pulling your navel back towards your spine, this is incorrect as it encourages you to pull your waist back. You have already learned the correct way to activate your pelvic floor and deep abdominal muscles (inner core), so persist with your correct activation.

Kate, 45 years, was referred by a friend after mentioning her problematic bladder. She related bladder urgency and frequency, and a vaginal bulge that had developed six months earlier. Kate has commenced a gym programme eight months earlier, as her DEXA scan showed lumbar osteopenia (this is early stage osteoporosis). Her gym programme was great for improving her bone density, but the last straw for her pelvic floor. On examination, Kate had a muscle pattern of bearing down on her pelvic floor, instead of tensioning upwards when she coughed or tried to tension her pelvic floor muscles. Adding weights and sit-ups added more internal downwards pressure which led to vaginal prolapse.

Kate put her gym membership on hold for six months. She changed to riding a seated stationary bike and swimming. After learning the correct pelvic floor tensioning, she progressed to pelvic floor strength exercises. Kate then recommenced at the gym with a seated weights programme, stretch band and Fitball exercises.

4. Stop Running if you Leak

If you leak when you run, then your pelvic floor is not strong enough to counteract the impact of your foot hitting the ground, plus the impact from above of intestines and pelvic organs pushing down. You may feel fine as you run, but you cannot see what is happening inside, as supporting tissue is stretched to failure point.

Change your exercise to walking, swimming or bike riding as you focus on learning correct pelvic floor tensioning and strengthening. Develop your strength with core exercise programmes that you continue throughout your life. You MAY find that you are able to return to running after five or six months of pelvic floor and deep abdominal strengthening.

If you return to running without any leaking after strengthening your pelvic floor and core, you must balance this activity with ongoing exercise to keep your core muscles strong.

Fig. 13 shows the effect of intra abdominal pressure when the pelvic floor muscles are weak or uncoordinated. The pelvic floor must tension upwards to resist this downward pressure.

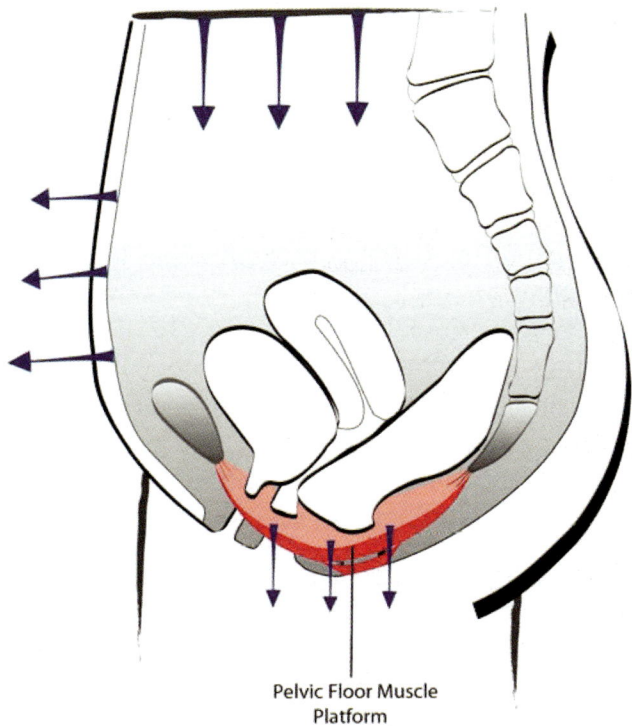

Pelvic Floor Muscle
Platform

When litfting or coughing, depression occurs if the Pelvic Floor and Transversus are weak and do not contract correctly. Their role is to tension up and hold.

Fig. 13 - Pelvic Floor Depression and Prolapse

□ **C a s e   S t u d y** □

Megan, a 32-year-old chiropractor, was referred for advice after delivering her second baby. She was slim and fit, and resumed running at 12 weeks post-birth. At six months, she returned to work part-time. She was still breastfeeding and her periods had not returned.

Megan was concerned because she leaked when she ran. She continued despite ongoing loss.

She needed much convincing to stop running and start walking instead. She correctly activated and strengthened her pelvic floor and used vaginal oestrogen pessaries.

After four months of strengthening, she was able to jog without any urine loss, but balanced this with Fitball exercises for core strength. Megan was highly motivated to maintain her pelvic floor strength exercises daily to prevent urine loss so she could continue jogging.

CAUTION

Do not expect to be able to automatically return to running after childbirth. Be flexible and prepared to change your type of exercise. For Megan, returning to running at 12 weeks before strengthening her pelvic floor was inviting more fascial tearing.

5. Don't Stop Exercising

Don't allow pelvic floor problems to stop you from doing some appropriate type of exercise. If you stop being active, then your muscles will weaken further, weight gain will be faster and you may become depressed. Abdominal weight gain, plus weakened pelvic floor muscles, will set the scene for future problems.

Change the type of activity so that your pelvic floor is not so stressed. When you swim, your body weight is supported by the water. When you sit down and ride a pushbike, your pelvic floor is supported from underneath. Try gentle Pilates and Fitball exercises, with a skilful, trained therapist, as these exercises focus on pelvic and deep abdominal muscle activation.

When lying on your back to exercise, stop any exercise that pushes your pelvic floor down and out or causes your abdomen to bulge upwards. This abdominal bulging is a sign that you need to go back and relearn your pelvic floor tensioning. Avoid curl-ups on a Fitball.

6. Lose Weight

Weight gain happens in two ways. Subcutaneous fat is deposited under the skin and visceral fat is laid down around your internal organs. The internal fat deposits are an extra weight down on your pelvic floor that weakened muscles will struggle to support.

Studies undertaken on moderately overweight women showed that a significant improvement in continence occurred when weight was lost. The improvement happened when they lost as little as 5% of their weight.[15]

Be sensible – forget the latest fad diet. Don't put any unrealistic pressure on yourself. Realise that weight loss is long term. It is about making permanent changes to what you eat, and adding regular exercise to your day.

Your body needs fruits, vegetables, lean protein, complex carbohydrates and good oil from nuts, fish and avocados. Join a weight loss support group, or visit your local dietician for a tailored eating plan that will become a lifetime way of eating. You can choose to swallow food without thinking of the effect it will have on your body OR you can make conscious choices to eat what your body needs on a daily basis.

Re-programme your brain to think about the foods that your body needs and avoid focusing on the foods that you know will fertilise fat cells.

Close your eyes and imagine, spread on a table, three to four pieces of fruit and five to seven serves of vegetables, two to three serves of protein, two to three serves of dairy, four to six serves of whole grain bread, high fibre cereal, nuts, rice, beans or pasta. This is what you are advised to eat every day. If you follow these guidelines, it does not leave a lot of room for fast food. Now try another check of how close your daily food intake is to the above list.

Combine sensible eating with some exercise EVERY DAY OF YOUR LIFE.

Keep exercising – just find the right type that suits you.

7. Become a Pelvic Floor Athlete

Do you know how athletes reach the top of their field? They rarely miss a day of training.

If you are serious about changing pelvic floor problems, then you need to exercise these muscles EVERY DAY. Adopt an athlete's mentality. The results will be achieved if you put in the work. I was speechless when I heard a Paralympic gold medal swimmer relate how he trained every day for four years to take half a second off his old world record. He even trained on Christmas Day. For me the lesson was, what you do *every* day is what counts, not just erratic bursts of activity.

How easy is it to clean your teeth? You don't even have to think about it – you just brush and floss your pearly whites twice a day. STICK with your pelvic floor exercises until they become an everyday routine. Women with incontinence have thinner pelvic floor muscles, but after a muscle training programme, the pelvic floor regains thickness.[16]

A pelvic floor athlete also uses ORGASM to strengthen. Yes, the high level of vaginal tensioning and contraction that orgasm produces is a brilliant workout for your pelvic floor. Remember, your training exercises will work to strengthen the intensity of your orgasm. A strong pelvic floor = a stronger orgasm. When you orgasm, your pelvic floor muscles can contact between five to 15 times at 0.8 second intervals.

□ **Case Study** □

Alice, a 28-year-old florist with a six-year-old, consulted me because of prolapse, bladder urgency and worsening constipation. She reported poor sensation with intercourse, and experienced only occasional mild orgasms. Prior to her daughter's birth, she was able to orgasm quickly with intense contractions. Alice had lost confidence sexually as her partner told her that he could not feel much sensation during intercourse. She had difficulty inserting a tampon (it often slipped out) and sometimes intercourse was painful, as her cervix had prolapsed down into her vagina. She regularly strained to empty her bowel. After standing all day, she reported vaginal heaviness. Her work involved lifting heavy buckets filled with water and flowers. She had started pelvic floor exercises but with no improvement to her symptoms.

When Alice activated her pelvic floor muscles, she incorrectly pushed down, which only aggravated her prolapse. Alice found it difficult to learn the correct pattern of tensioning initially, as she had to change her old muscle pattern of bearing down. By her third visit, she proudly demonstrated how she had learned correct pelvic floor tensioning, and reported less bladder urgency. She had learned to open her bowel without straining, and had started a regular walking programme.

After progressing to strength exercises, she had fewer episodes of intercourse pain and pressure sensations from prolapse at the end of the day. She was able to tension up her pelvic floor when standing and lifting. Alice reduced the amount of water in the buckets that she lifted at work.

Her proudest achievement though, was her reconnection with her pelvic floor and the heightened sensation with orgasm.

8. Back off at Period Time

In the week before menstruation, you may experience PMT and less bladder control along with vaginal heaviness. Uterine cramping and sacroiliac joint aching can develop at the start of your period. These are related to variable hormonal levels and sometimes to pelvic floor muscle weakness. Do you feel these symptoms, ignore them anyway and push yourself physically? This is crazy – listen to your body, and try being kinder to yourself.

Use this time to get some rest and regeneration. Back off your workload. Try an easy Pilates or yoga class or go for a walk instead of 'punishing' your body at the gym. When you are physically exhausted, tense and irritable, your menstrual symptoms will be aggravated. Some quiet, self-reflective time will help restore your emotional and physical strength prior to the start of another monthly cycle.

9. Teach your Daughters

If your daughters grow up seeing you tired, stressed, cranky and refusing to rest (while you frantically care for everyone else), they get the message that it is important for a woman to place everyone else's needs before her own. They in turn may learn this same pattern and feel they have no alternative but to push themselves when they should back off.

When your daughters (and sons) graduate from the 'potty' to using an adult sized toilet, it is ESSENTIAL that they have a high stool for support under their feet. This is vital to stop them from falling into the toilet and to prevent slumping and straining to open their bowel. Due to poor food choices today, children are more prone to constipation. Without a high stool, they tend to slump and strongly pull their waist back as they bear down with straining. This may make them more prone to emptying problems, urinary incontinence, and pelvic floor or abdominal muscle imbalance problems.

10. Control Urgency

Don't obey every signal your bladder sends you. Learn to put off voiding until you have at least 250-300mls in your bladder. The Golden Rule is to empty your bladder only five or six times a day.

Give up artificial sweeteners, as some will markedly aggravate bladder urgency and frequency. They can cause more bowel wind and soft motions. If you are experiencing urgency, give up caffeine – coffee, tea, soft drinks with caffeine, Diet Colas and chocolate (sorry, but it does contain caffeine). Remember that green tea also contains caffeine. Alcohol relaxes your bladder, so you may have an unexpected loss of urine when you laugh or walk. Nicotine also aggravates urgency.

You often hear that urgency is 'all in your head'. Well, that's not totally correct. You do need to firmly command your bladder if you have recently passed urine and it starts to become urgent again. To gain lasting control over urgency, learn to correctly tension and then strengthen your pubococcygeus muscle. This is the muscle that tensions the urethral sphincters and closes the sphincter at the base of your bladder (the action you learned in Putting it all Together, page 37).

Is your medication aggravating your bladder frequency, urgency, hesitancy or urinary retention? Ask your pharmacist to print out an information sheet about your medication, and read the side effects section. Then ask your doctor to review your medication if side effects include bladder problems.

Keep drinking water. Many women with urgency and frequency markedly restrict their fluid intake to control urine loss. This can cause more bladder urgency, tiredness, dehydration and constipation.

The Pelvic Floor throughout Life and Activity

The Young Pelvic Floor

Most bladder and bowel problems in children require medical review. Clinicians and researchers are realising that some problems that present in the adult pelvic floor started with childhood habits. Becoming aware of which habits cause problems will help you talk to your children about changing the damaging habits. Patterns of toileting learned in childhood stay with the child for life.

Important Tip

> **Ask your children how often they empty their bladder and bowel each day.**

Listen to your children if they say, 'But I don't need to do a wee'.

Children should empty their bladder when they get the urge, and not when it suits the parent. Forcing a partially full bladder to empty teaches the bladder that it is all right to frequently pass smaller amounts of urine. Encourage children to drink at least four glasses of water a day (as well as other fluids) and ensure they empty their bladder about four or five times a day.

They might say, 'I hate the school toilets – they smell'.

Ask children how often they empty their bladder at school. If a child drinks correctly, they should empty their bladder once or twice at school. Some children will go to the toilet but refuse to wee because of smells, noise, self-consciousness or lack of toilet paper. They walk around with urgency (due to a full bladder), but hold the bladder sphincter clamped shut. This can cause leaking, wet pants and ongoing urgency as the bladder contracts.

If the child hurries bladder emptying and anxiously sits on the toilet with their waist tightly pulled in, their bladder sphincter does not fully relax. This can lead to a problem with pelvic floor muscle co-ordination, which may cause wet pants initially and problem bladder emptying as they mature. Teach children to relax their tummy forwards to empty their bladder fully and to sit until the urine flow finishes. If the bladder does not fully empty, it can cause bladder infections. NEVER tell a child to push down to empty their bladder.

Research is now connecting a higher rate of urinary incontinence in adult women to their childhood voiding problems.[17] Pelvic floor physiotherapists report an association between childhood daytime wetting, ongoing bedwetting, urgency and prolonged coughing (asthma), with urge incontinence in adult years.

Perhaps the child says, 'My poo is too hard to push out'.

This indicates that your child may not be drinking enough water. Soft drinks and frozen drinks often contain caffeine, which draws water out of the body (diuretic).

It could indicate that they do not eat enough fibre rich foods. Children today are permitted more choice over what they eat. As they are not able to reason with a mature brain, they will eat for taste, making low fibre choices from fast food, candy, chips and biscuits. For healthy bowel function, they require fruit or vegetables with most meals, and unrefined grains (multigrain or rye bread, full oats porridge). This gives the correct fibre and intestinal flora for a normal, soft, easy-to-pass bowel motion. Remember that children cannot be expected to make correct food choices – they need guidance, however unpopular that makes the parent.

When a child starts sitting on the 'big toilet', their spine and bottom will slump down into the toilet if they have no support under their feet. Children must rest their feet on a high stool so they can sit up straight. Without foot support, they round their spine into a C curve, pull their tummy back and strain down into their bottom. This position and action close the anal sphincter, making emptying much more difficult.

Teach children to sit up tall on the toilet, feet on the stool, and then fully relax their tummy forwards as their bowel opens. This will teach them the correct method of emptying throughout their life.

Teach girls to wipe from front to back to prevent E. coli bacteria from entering the urethra and causing infection.

Ask children how often they poo. More children are now visiting their doctor or emergency department with strong tummy pain. When the abdomen is x-rayed, it can show a backup of faeces through the intestine as the bowel may not have opened for up to a week.

Constipation is another cause of wet pants during the day for a child, due to the pressure on the bladder from the build-up of faeces.

The child may say, 'I wet my pants when I laugh or jump'.

Some girls lose urine when they giggle and others while running and jumping.

If bladder and kidney ultrasounds are clear, then the problem may be due to a muscular imbalance. Many sports teach children to firmly brace their abdomen by pulling their waist back. If this becomes a constant strong muscle pattern, the child will be over-developing their outer tummy muscles at the expense of the inner postural muscles that support the spine and pelvic floor. Teach children from an early age how to relax their waist and then tension their pelvic floor and deep abdominal muscles.

An easy way is to have them pretend to attach a 'tail' to their coccyx (show them where this is). Ask them to sit upright, breathe out and release their tummy forwards.

When they breathe out next time, keep their tummy soft and tell them to slowly (in their mind) draw their 'tail' forwards and slowly, gently, lift it up between their legs. Hold and breathe. Done correctly, this will tension up the pelvic floor and not the buttock and waist muscles. If your child can learn and continue this correct muscle pattern in childhood, they will have learnt the pattern for life.

This can be difficult to learn, so seek expert guidance from a pelvic floor physiotherapist.

□ **Case Study** □

Madeline

Madeline, eight years, was referred for advice, as she was losing urine at callisthenics classes, four days a week, and when she laughed. Every day she strained hard to empty her bowel, sitting on the toilet in a slumped position. She sat bolt upright on the treatment table with her tummy firmly drawn back. She had learned this muscle pattern from three years of training and regular competition callisthenics.

After some time and encouragement, Madeline was able to sit upright (with a high stool under her feet), while releasing her super strong little tummy forwards. She was taught how to sit correctly on the toilet and relax her tummy to empty her bowel, and how to correctly tension her pelvic and deep abdominal muscles during the day, and before doing her callisthenics. Her mum agreed to supervise more regular water intake, provide more fibre rich meals and snacks and purchase a high stool for toileting.

Four weeks later, Madeline returned to relate that her bowel opened daily without straining (relaxed tummy) and that over the

59

previous few weeks she had had no urine loss. She was able to tension her pelvic floor effectively before jumping and laughing. This daily tensioning reinforced the correct action in her brain.

Bedwetting

Around 10% of seven year olds wet the bed at night and 2 to 3% during the day. This declines in adolescents. Children with delayed school entry and handicaps have a 25% rate of bedwetting.[18] Many pelvic floor physiotherapists specialise in treating childhood incontinence.

For more information and suggested treatment of bedwetting, go to www.continence.org.au

A study of Canadian teenage secondary school girls shows self-reported daytime urge incontinence in 17% of the girls and stress incontinence in 15%.[19]

These girls have a higher risk of more severe pelvic floor dysfunction following childbirth and menopause. Teenage incontinence issues should not be accepted. Earlier treatment is needed to avoid more significant pelvic floor problems in adult years.

Sport and the Pelvic Floor

There is a high rate of stress and urge urine loss in elite female athletes. Stress loss occurs while running, jumping or sneezing. Urgency occurs when your bladder suddenly contracts, which can cause urine loss. One researcher reports that 28% of elite athletes lose urine while playing their sport.[20] Another reports a 52% loss in athletes and dancers during their sport.[21] None of the athletes in these studies had given birth. Athletes with an eating disorder have significantly higher rates of stress and urge incontinence than athletes with normal eating patterns.[22]

If elite athletes have this loss of bladder control, then what is it like for the majority of women who play sport? High impact activities such as running, landing and jumping result in higher rates of urine loss. Low impact activities such as golf result in less urine loss. If a woman becomes distressed due to poor bladder control then she is more likely to stop her sport, often giving other reasons for stopping. Problems then start with weight gain and loss of muscle strength and bulk as fat replaces muscle. Weight gain is one of the main predictors of future prolapse. Other women will persist with activity, using tampons and vaginal pessary supports to stop urine loss by supporting up under the bladder neck. If you have a vaginal bladder neck support in place, this is the time to focus on effective pelvic floor strength exercises. Change your activity if you leak, but don't stop exercising.

Remember the role of your pelvic floor? The muscular sling not only supports your pelvic organs from downward pressure inside your abdomen, but also tensions to close the sphincters that keep you continent. A strong pelvic floor that will correctly tension and hold when you jump, run or dance is your first line of defence against urine loss. If you cannot stop urine loss with high impact activities (after a strengthening programme), then change your sport or activity.

Our society places a lot of emphasis on exercise. The role of pelvic floor exercises and suitable types of training needs to be considered in order to prevent pelvic floor damage in young women. I am convinced that females need to train differently from males. New research is needed to look at the effects of training and exercise prescription on the pelvic floor in girls and young female athletes.

If a girl is trained to over-strengthen her outer abdominals with constant strong waist tension, inappropriate sit-ups, medicine ball rotations and double leg lifts, then she learns to create regular inner pressure down on her pelvic floor. If she does not know how to tension her pelvic floor, learns an uncoordinated pattern, has weak muscles or uses an action that bears down, then damage is promoted. Other young women are not able to relax a tightly held pelvic floor – this in turn will cause weakness.

Coaches and trainers need education to replace damaging abdominal routines with exercises that emphasise deep abdominal and pelvic floor strengthening. Body holds, balancing exercises with added weights or stretch bands, Fitball holds, Pilates and yoga poses are suitable activities when training abdominal muscles in young girls, teenagers and women. Any athlete's control in their sport will be improved when their core muscles are stronger. Young female athletes need to know whether they can correctly tension their pelvic floor, or if they are incorrectly substituting the strong outer abdominal muscles that cause more internal pressure down on the pelvic floor.

Screening programs that identify the girls and women who substitute incorrect abdominal muscles for their pelvic floor muscles must be a priority with medical and sporting groups, if they are serious about changing pelvic floor dysfunction in female athletes.

Emphasis on strengthening the outer abdominals will lead to strengthening the very muscles that cause a strong downward pressure on the pelvic floor. Our body (and brain) learns that these dominant muscles are the ones to use when tensioning the pelvic floor. This pattern is then repeated throughout life and will inevitably lead to pelvic floor problems.

Athletes with hyperactive pelvic floor muscles will benefit from learning abdominal and pelvic floor relaxation before correctly coordinating these muscles.

Teenage girls and women in their twenties and thirties can get de-conditioned pelvic floor muscles. Lack of specific exercise will cause the vaginal muscles to thin. When a woman with a deconditioned pelvic floor becomes pregnant, supporting a heavy uterus is more difficult. After childbirth, weak pelvic floor muscles don't recover as quickly and often struggle to support the pelvic organs. This can lead to dropping or prolapse of the pelvic organs, lower back pain and discomfort during intercourse.

Pregnancy and the Pelvic Floor

Don't leave it until pregnancy to find your pelvic floor muscles. Ideally, you want strong effective pelvic floor muscles before becoming pregnant.

If you are incontinent before pregnancy, then you are five times more likely to leak after birth than women who are continent before pregnancy.[23]

Urinary incontinence during pregnancy roughly doubles the likelihood of urinary incontinence at three months post baby. This is regardless of whether the delivery is vaginal or by Caesarean section.[24]

Just the weight of your baby during pregnancy can weaken and strain your pelvic floor. However, studies show that pelvic floor exercises during pregnancy will decrease post-birth urinary incontinence. Yet in a Norwegian study of 467 women, only a few did regular pelvic floor exercises during pregnancy.[25]

As your pregnancy progresses, your pelvic floor and deep abdominal muscles are called upon more and more to support the growing load of baby and fluid.

Many women experience some degree of discomfort or pain from stretching of internal supporting ligaments, sciatic pain in their buttock or leg, pubic symphysis and sacroiliac joint pain, or in their mid spine and chest. Some may experience a separation of their outer tummy muscles. Others develop an increased curve in their lower back that causes low backache.

How severely you suffer with musculoskeletal pain during pregnancy is related to the strength and support that your pelvic floor and deep abdominal muscles provide. These muscles support the weight of your enlarged uterus and work to keep your lower back in a neutral position, so you don't develop an increased curve in your lower back, which causes lower back pain. Learn to hold your spine with a normal curve as you walk, by gently tilting your buttocks under.

Researchers who looked at pregnant women with lower back pain found that 52% had pelvic floor dysfunction. Successful treatment of lower back pain in pregnancy should also focus on correct activation of pelvic floor and co-ordination with other core muscles.[26]

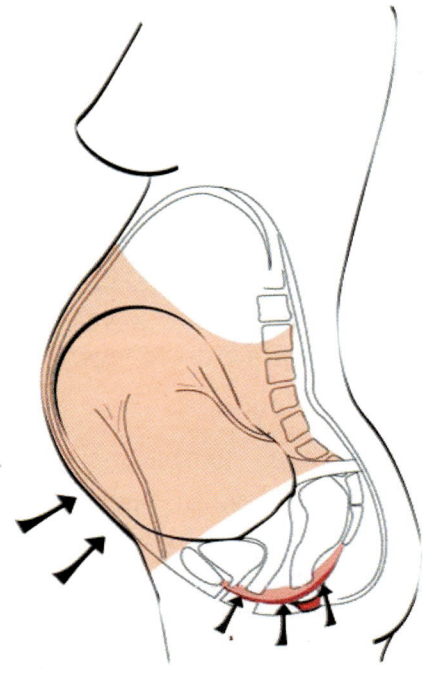

This muscular corset supports the growing uterus to prevent pain in the spine, sacroiliac joints and groin.

Fig. 14 - Pelvic Floor and Transversus Provide Support for the Pregnant Uterus

As pregnancy progresses, some women suffer with worsening pain due to Pelvic Instability. This is primarily caused by lack of activation and support from the inner core of muscles. Intense pain can be felt in the lower back, sacroiliac joints, buttocks, pubic symphysis and groin, making it difficult to walk and change positions. Many women find that wearing a sacroiliac support belt or an abdominal support helps to control the pain. Your first step towards reducing these symptoms is to learn to activate your pelvic floor and deep abdominal muscles correctly, as outlined earlier in this book.

To learn more about pelvic instability and treatment, visit www.pelvicinstability.org.au

Choose upright chairs that support your lower back and discourage you from slumping. Avoid sitting on the floor if you have sacroiliac or lower back pain. Put a support or pillow in your car to keep the small curve in your lower back. Wear low-heeled shoes and avoid sitting with crossed legs.

Exercise during Pregnancy

If you have exercised regularly before pregnancy, then you should be able to continue that exercise, but will need to modify the intensity. The hormone relaxin softens pelvic joints prior to delivery, so it doesn't make sense to exercise as hard as you did before pregnancy. During pregnancy, it is vitally important to exercise your inner core of supporting muscles correctly, as well as your strength muscles.

Exercise during pregnancy can help prepare you for childbirth by building endurance in your supporting muscles, making it easier for you to counteract your body's changing centre of gravity. Ideal exercise gets your heart pumping, stretches muscles, manages weight gain and helps you prepare for labour. Good activities include walking, swimming, yoga, dancing, Fitball, Tai Chi, light weights and gentle exercise classes. Be sure to learn the correct pelvic floor tensioning before you start any exercise programme.

The physiotherapy departments of most large hospital run pre- and post-baby exercise classes, so call your local hospital to find out class availability and times.

For a physiotherapist-designed pregnancy and post-baby workout, visit www.preggiebellies.com.au

When pregnant, remember to:

- Avoid heavy weights, especially lifting overhead
- Stretch before and after exercise, but not excessively
- Stop if you start to feel tired or fatigued. Don't overdo any activity
- After six months, avoid lying on your back to exercise
- Stay cool, and drink plenty of water
- Avoid sit-ups or curl-ups.

Important Tip

Sit upright on a Fitball at your computer, during and after pregnancy. Your deep abdominal and pelvic floor muscles will be activated to keep you upright and balanced on the ball.

While you are sitting, take a work break and balance with one foot off the floor while you slowly move both arms overhead. Keep control of your hips and trunk as your arms move.

Aerobic exercise is not advised if you have:

- high blood pressure
- incompetent cervix

- premature labour

- pre-term rupture of membranes or leaking fluid

- dizziness, cramping

- severe joint pain

- shortness of breath

- vaginal bleeding or uterine contractions

- a sudden swelling of ankles, feet or hands.

To view guidelines for exercise during pregnancy, visit www.sma.org.au/pdfdocuments/Fact_sheet_2.pdf

Birth and the Pelvic Floor

How a woman gives birth and which interventions are used during birth play a major role in pelvic floor function after birth. Recently, two of my clients delivered in the same week. While one chose a home-based birth with no medical intervention, the other mum was adamant about delivering with an elective C-section in a major hospital. Every method of birthing has benefits and complications. Culture, family, socio-economic factors, age and education all influence the way a woman chooses to give birth. Knowledge about birthing is essential for women to take an informed role in their birthing process.

Start with exploring what happens in the majority of problem-free births. In antenatal or birthing classes, the focus should be on how to optimise the birthing experience rather than what can go wrong.

To attend childbirth classes, contact:

- the Childbirth Education Association in your state

- your state Physiotherapy Association for Physiotherapist run classes; or

- click onto www.birthinternational.com

Childbirth is widely recognised as one of the main causes of pelvic floor dysfunction. The factors that increase the risk of pelvic floor damage with birth and ongoing problems after birth are:

- poor birthing positions
- forced pushing with a closed epiglottis
- instrumental delivery, vacuum extraction
- third- and fourth-degree perineal tears
- a second stage longer than two hours
- delivering your first baby
- your baby weighing over 4000 grams
- epidural anaesthesia
- episiotomy
- poor connective tissue[27]

The International Continence Society reports that, 'Over the course of a lifetime, one in 30,000 Scandinavian women die in pregnancy or labour. For a woman from Africa, the risk is one in 12. However, for every woman who dies in labour in the developing world, many more find their lives destroyed by terrible injuries because of untreated obstructed labour. The developed world is only now becoming aware of the devastation to women's lives, largely because women in the developing world have no voice in the international community'.[28] For women in the developing world, the emphasis must be on programmes to access medical screening and interventions to prevent the high loss of life and injury. Women in the Western world are able to focus on optimal birthing positions, minimal interventions and maximising their birthing experience.

Important Tip

Before birthing, talk to your doctor or midwife about the routine use of interventions that can increase the risk of pelvic floor disorders.[29]

Ask your doctor or midwife about birthing positions and options that can lessen pelvic floor damage. If your delivery is proceeding well, avoid lying on your back to deliver as this prevents your sacrum from moving during delivery. If your sacrum cannot move during vaginal delivery (second stage), this will increase your risk of having an episiotomy. A review of 177 research papers shows that, 'The routine use of episiotomy to prevent severe perineal tears, urinary incontinence, faecal incontinence and genital prolapse should be abandoned'.[30]

Unnecessary cutting prior to your baby's head being delivered can lead to more severe tearing. Cutting and stitching through the pelvic floor muscles leads to atrophy (muscle wasting) and weakness in the pelvic floor.

Choose side lying, upright squatting with your thighs and buttocks supported on a birthing cushion, or kneeling. Talk to your midwife about alternative positions or a water birth. If you are sedated, too tired or need an instrumental delivery then a recumbent position is chosen.

The researchers who looked at how women are birthed and then related this to their subsequent pelvic floor problems, state, 'At least some of the less desirable outcomes attributed to vaginal births have been due to obstetric practices that are in need of improvement. Routine and overuse of episiotomy, routine use of epidurals, prolonged closed glottis pushing, lithotomy and other non-physiologic positions for birth all will cause differential increases for vaginal birth in the very perineal and pelvic floor problems to which this review has been directed. If these and other obstetric practices were improved, the reported differences between vaginal birth and caesarean section pelvic floor outcomes would likely narrow substantially'.

Women who deliver through an intact pelvic floor are less likely to suffer with vaginal pain during intercourse. Women who birth with episiotomy, significant tears and the use of forceps or suction, report a higher frequency and severity of pain with intercourse at six months post-birth.[31]

Women who birth vaginally have a higher rate of stress incontinence and vaginal prolapse than C-section women, because of the increased chance of muscle, connective tissue and nerve damage sustained as the baby's head engages the pelvic floor. Research shows that when major muscle damage occurs with vaginal childbirth, this is associated with vaginal prolapse.[32] These studies did not look at the birthing positions or what interventions were used. When adverse outcomes are minimised, then women will start to view vaginal births more positively.

If you have hypermobile joints (connective tissue problems) and a family history of prolapse, then you are definitely more at risk of prolapse with vaginal birth[33] and should ask your obstetrician's advice about a C-section delivery.

For more information about preventing pelvic floor dysfunction when giving birth, visit www.childbirthconnection.org/article.asp?ck=10208

Women who choose to deliver by an elective Caesarean section minimise the risk of major muscle damage and tearing. However, the likelihood of urge incontinence after the age of 50 is no different between those who have had a C-section and those who have undergone a vaginal delivery. A C-section delivery is no guarantee of a problem-free pelvic floor. Studies show that the prevalence of stress or urge incontinence and intravaginal prolapse was 42% in women with one or more vaginal deliveries, as opposed to 35% in women who had had C-section deliveries.[34] Women who are in labour prior to the decision to perform a C-section sustain more pelvic floor problems than women who elect to birth by a C-section delivery.

With a C-section, your deep abdominal muscle is cut, so after delivery it's important to check that this muscle is activating correctly (with your pelvic floor) and that, once healing has occurred, you commence a strengthening programme for your deep abdominal as well as pelvic floor muscles.

After a C-section, some women report loss of sensation around their abdominal incision line, and don't know how to contract their deep abdominal muscle, causing a loss of control over their lower abdomen. This loss of control and strength in the deep abdominal muscle leads to a slack abdomen and an increased risk of lower back pain and pelvic floor problems.

To learn more about a Caesarean section delivery, visit www.canaustralia.net

□ Case Study □

Maria, 38 years, had delivered her only child by C-section four years earlier. She related increasing episodes of lower back pain and worsening bladder urgency over the past three years. She had not done any pelvic floor exercises pre- or post-birth. She was not able to flatten her slack lower tummy and had less feeling around her incision line. She stopped exercising because of her bulging abdomen and gained even more weight. Her bowel function had slowed and she strained to open her bowel because of constipation.

On examination, Maria had lost the ability to tension her pelvic floor and deep abdominal muscle corset. Her pelvic floor had started to descend and this left her pelvic organs with poor support when she lifted or coughed. Her spine was at risk of injury, as the inner muscular corset did not contract effectively to protect her spine when lifting or sneezing.

After learning to locate and tension her pelvic floor and deep abdominal muscles, Maria lost her bladder urgency. After working on a strength programme for four months, she was able to tension her deep abdominal and pelvic floor with all daily activities and reported no episodes of lower back pain. (It became automatic for Maria to tension when she was active). She changed her bowel straining (by adding more fibre, water and new position) which lessened the downward strain on her pelvic floor.

Post-Baby Pelvic Floor

Congratulations. It's time to laugh, be in awe and celebrate the incredible arrival of the divine little person that you have created. It's also time to thank your body for the marathon effort of giving birth.

Initially euphoric, then exhausted, it's normal that you turn your attention to your baby, whose arrival has turned your regular daily schedule upside down.

This is the most important time in your life

to pay attention to your pelvic floor

Your pelvic floor muscles may be tender and swollen if you sustained any tearing, or had an episiotomy, stitches or other interventions. You may have a painful abdomen after a c-section delivery. If you sustained any bruising, tearing or cutting, your pelvic floor will need intense rehabilitation. You are told, 'Don't forget your pelvic floor exercises', but find that you have great difficulty locating the right muscles, or they just don't seem to tighten and hold in the same way as before giving birth.

Start gently tensioning 24 hours after birth (vaginal) and continue a strengthening programme for at least six months. Then continue a maintenance pelvic floor exercise programme throughout your life.

If you had an easier delivery with no pelvic floor damage, take time to focus on your pelvic floor muscles. Remember that your newborn will soon grow to be a heavy toddler. If you decide to have another baby, your pelvic floor has to support the weight of your growing baby, as well as the load of your heavy toddler who demands to be lifted and carried on your hip. So reconnect with your pelvic floor soon after giving birth and continue these exercises EVERY DAY OF YOUR LIFE.

This is the time to see your pelvic floor physiotherapist to:

1. **CONTROL** swelling and pain. Ice reduces swelling and a thick pad placed inside firm stretchy briefs will help control swelling. Any pain or swelling prevents your pelvic floor from contracting normally.

2. **PREVENT** straining with bowel emptying.

   If you bear down on recently torn or stitched pelvic/vaginal tissue, then you will do more damage, and possibly cause prolapse. Protect your pelvic floor by firmly holding a pad up over the front of your pelvic floor (vaginal area) as your bowel opens. Use the bowel opening position described in Ten Healthy Habits for the Pelvic Floor (page 40). Stay relaxed around your waist and abdomen. Straining increases your risk of developing haemorrhoids. Long-term straining of the bowel can lead to rectal or anal sphincter prolapse as well as vaginal prolapse.

   Be aware that any pain-relieving medication can cause constipation post-birth.

   You may need prunes, fibre or a suppository so that your bowel opens easily without straining. Avoid laxatives that contain senna. PLEASE ask your midwife for help if you are constipated or cannot open your bowel without straining. Focus on foods that are rich in dietary fibre – fruit, vegetables, beans, lentils and whole grains. This is not only important for your fibre intake, but also to provide the best nutrition in your milk for breast-feeding.

For more information on treating constipation, visit www.aboutconstipation.org/characteristics.html

Anal sphincter tears that cause incontinence are often not detected following delivery.[35]

One study showed that 10.7% of first mums at six weeks post-birth had an anal sphincter tear.[36] Another showed that there was a higher rate of post-birth anal incontinence in women who were older and who had hypermobile joints and large babies.[37] Because of embarrassment, many women do not seek treatment or further investigation of anal incontinence. This incontinence rarely 'goes away' by itself, so visit your obstetrician and pelvic floor physiotherapist for ongoing management.

Pelvic floor physiotherapists work in private practices, community clinics and large hospitals. You don't need a referral to see a physiotherapist in private practice. Many large hospitals have a specialist women's physiotherapy outpatient section where you can receive assessment, treatment and management advice.

3. **LEARN** how to tension your pelvic floor muscles CORRECTLY. After birth, your pelvic floor muscles do not always automatically start working again correctly. Many women report that it 'just does not feel the same as before delivery.' In a 2004 study, the women who started their exercises early post-birth were drier than those who did not start their exercises.[38] How soon do you need to start pelvic floor exercises post-birth? Take 24 hours rest then start gently tensioning your pelvic floor.

75

Learn deep abdominal and pelvic floor tensioning before lifting or coughing. If you leave hospital without knowing how to tension your pelvic floor correctly, then make an appointment to see a pelvic floor physiotherapist after you return home. Do not forget about this most important area of your body in the busy post-birth time.

4. **START** a training programme to build strength and endurance in your pelvic floor. This needs to be monitored and progressed at regular intervals until you and your physiotherapist are satisfied with your strength. From now on, you must tension your pelvic floor EVERY DAY OF YOUR LIFE, before you lift, cough or sneeze or before you start any exercise. Repeat this tensioning until it becomes an automatic behaviour (like brushing your teeth).

   If you developed an increased curve in your lower back during pregnancy, now's the time to regain your normal lower back curve. Practise sitting with your weight over your sitting bones and lift up your sternum. Practise your pelvic floor and deep abdominal tensioning as you maintain this posture. Then stand, again with sternum lifted, and waist relaxed. As you breathe out, slowly tension your pelvic and deep abdominal muscles. Learn to hold this position as you walk and prevent your pelvis from dropping forwards. Keep these same muscles engaged when you bend over to change or lift up your baby.

Important Tip

If you only do your pelvic floor exercises in sitting, then you will not effectively strengthen. It's crucial to progress your exercises to standing, then walking, squatting and finally when lifting a weight.

You perform these movements every day, so your pelvic floor needs to be able to keep up with the rest of your active muscles. If you cannot tension your pelvic floor when you stand up and cough, then how can your pelvic floor stay tensioned when you squat down and pick up a heavy toddler?

Post-Birth Rules

1. Never Lift or Push More than your Pelvic Floor Can Resist

If you feel your pelvic floor pushes down when you do any activity (e.g. when you pick up a child), then your pelvic floor is not engaging or is not strong enough and you are promoting prolapse. The 12 weeks after birth are when you are most in danger of prolapse. Some of the young mums who attend my clinic report that their prolapse suddenly happened after straining with constipation, moving house, lifting older children, returning to farm work, returning to the gym or as a result of prolonged coughing due to a chest infection.

2. Watch out for the Blues

If your periods have not started because of ongoing breastfeeding, your oestrogen levels will be lower. This can cause decreased libido and vaginal dryness, so a lubricant with help with intercourse. Hormonal imbalances post partum can contribute to incontinence, constipation and post-natal depression.

For more information about post-baby blues and depression, visit: www.beyondblue.org.au/postnataldepression/

3. Make Time to Rehabilitate your Pelvic Floor

Ideally allow between 18 months and two years to re-strengthen your body between babies. When pregnancies are close together, your pelvic floor may not be strong enough to support the weight of another heavy uterus. Just the weight of your pregnancy can strain and weaken your pelvic floor, even before you deliver. Remember that during your second or third pregnancy, you have a toddler to pick up and carry as well. This adds up to a heavier load on your pelvic floor.

□ **Case Study** □

Robyn, 32 years old, called me to ask for advice. She was distressed, as she had just finished an 'ab buster' class, and had turned a minor outer tummy muscle separation (caused by pregnancy) into a major separation.

Robyn had done gym work with weights, 'pump' classes and a punishing abdominal routine for 10 years before her first pregnancy. After her first C-section baby, she developed bladder urgency. Six months after her second large baby was delivered by C-section, she returned to the gym to regain her fitness and control her tummy. After she had done 30 minutes of hard abdominal crunches, her outer tummy muscle (rectus abdominis) separated more below her navel and upwards towards her sternum.

When Robyn lay on her back and lifted her head forwards, her mid tummy spread open to a 3½-finger width separation.

Initially, she had no ability to tension her pelvic floor and deep abdominal muscles. When she attempted a pelvic floor contraction, her rectus abdominis and obliques contracted, causing a widening of the outer tummy tear. Robyn had no awareness of her pelvic floor, which did not tension and hold.

Over the next four months, Robyn correctly activated and strengthened her deep abdominal and pelvic floor muscles, avoided any sit-up movement and stopped lifting any more than her baby. The outer tummy muscle separation reduced to 1½-finger widths. She reported no further bladder urgency.

A wide separation that does not reduce may need surgical correction. It is not the actual muscle that splits, but the fascia that joins the sections of the muscle. The same tearing of the outer abdominal fascia that happens during pregnancy can also occur in your pelvic floor fascia. (This allows vaginal walls to sag).

Important Tip

> **Forget sit-ups during pregnancy and after birth. Find the correct muscles to flatten your tummy.**

This is essential if you have separated your outer abdominal muscle, or have any prolapse symptoms or urine loss. If you focus on sit-ups, then you risk further tearing and widening of the rectus diastasis. Focus on correct pelvic floor and deep abdominal activation, then progressive strengthening of these deep muscles. Studies show that menopausal women with an outer tummy muscle separation have more pelvic floor dysfunction than women with no separation[39], so rehabilitate your pelvic floor to prevent this future problem.

Remember, these inner core muscles are the ones that FLATTEN YOUR TUMMY. In sitting and standing, use these core muscles to flatten your tummy, and do not pull back at the waist as this pushes down on your pelvic floor.

(See Gym and the Pelvic Floor, page 91, for returning to the gym for 'at risk women'.)

Guidelines for Return to Activity

While some women have good pelvic floor control at six to eight weeks post-birth, others may still be struggling with weakness and symptoms of prolapse at six months. Remember that it takes up to four months for the effects of relaxin to pass. The hormone relaxin, causes your ligaments to soften during pregnancy in preparation for birthing.

The guidelines on the following page apply once you have learned correct pelvic floor and deep abdominal tensioning.

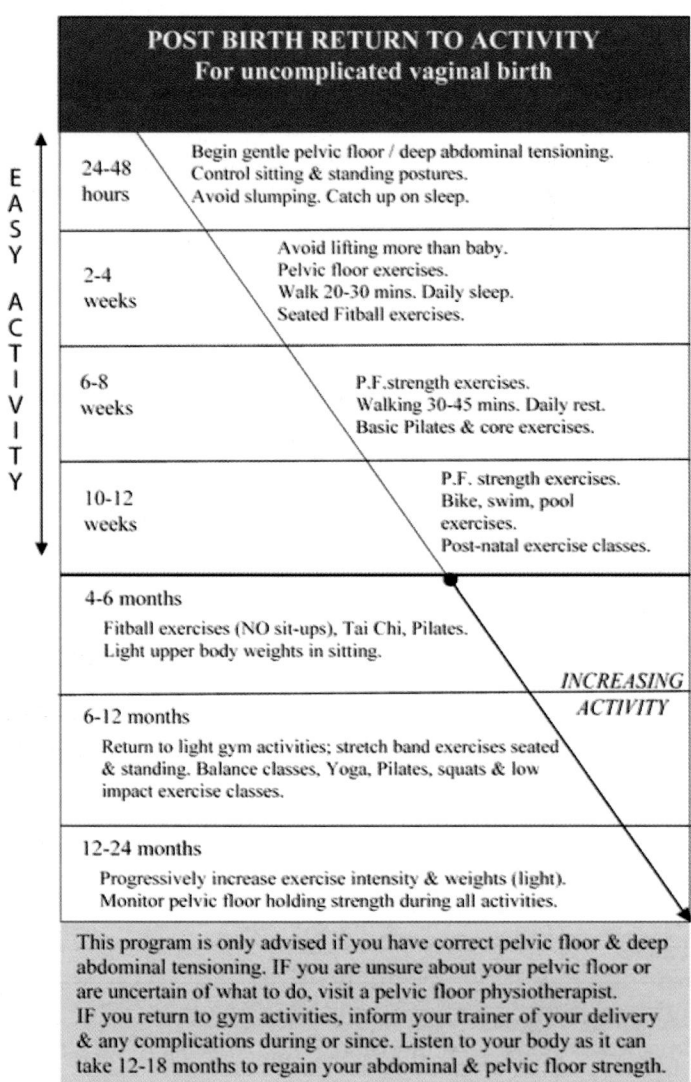

POST BIRTH RETURN TO ACTIVITY
For uncomplicated vaginal birth

EASY ACTIVITY

24-48 hours	Begin gentle pelvic floor / deep abdominal tensioning. Control sitting & standing postures. Avoid slumping. Catch up on sleep.
2-4 weeks	Avoid lifting more than baby. Pelvic floor exercises. Walk 20-30 mins. Daily sleep. Seated Fitball exercises.
6-8 weeks	P.F.strength exercises. Walking 30-45 mins. Daily rest. Basic Pilates & core exercises.
10-12 weeks	P.F. strength exercises. Bike, swim, pool exercises. Post-natal exercise classes.

4-6 months
Fitball exercises (NO sit-ups), Tai Chi, Pilates.
Light upper body weights in sitting.

INCREASING ACTIVITY

6-12 months
Return to light gym activities; stretch band exercises seated & standing. Balance classes, Yoga, Pilates, squats & low impact exercise classes.

12-24 months
Progressively increase exercise intensity & weights (light).
Monitor pelvic floor holding strength during all activities.

This program is only advised if you have correct pelvic floor & deep abdominal tensioning. IF you are unsure about your pelvic floor or are uncertain of what to do, visit a pelvic floor physiotherapist. IF you return to gym activities, inform your trainer of your delivery & any complications during or since. Listen to your body as it can take 12-18 months to regain your abdominal & pelvic floor strength.

Fig. 15 – Guidelines for returning to activity after birth

□ **Case Study** □

Trudy had delivered her third baby six months earlier. No one offered any advice when she said that she 'felt like everything was going to fall out'. (This should have set off alarm bells about imminent prolapse). Trudy was lifting her heavy two year old and occasionally her five year old. She had no idea of correct pelvic floor tensioning and used a strong waist bracing action, which increased the 'something falling out' sensation. She had tried playing tennis but stopped due to the 'scary' sensation.

Trudy learned correct pelvic floor and deep abdominal tensioning, lifted only her baby and avoided any bowel straining. At her second visit, she reported no prolapse sensation and over the next five months progressively strengthened her pelvic floor before returning to social tennis twice a week.

After Caesarean Section or Pelvic Surgery

- Support your incision line when moving or coughing.

- Start gentle pelvic floor tensioning after your stitches are removed (after pelvic surgery, start when catheter is removed).

- Do not lift more than your baby in the first six weeks. Plan to have help at home.

- Rest when your baby sleeps.

- After two to three weeks, start walking for 20 to 30 minutes, without a pram. Avoid hills. By the end of six to eight weeks, aim to walk for up to 30 to 40 minutes.

- At eight to 10 weeks, start exercises at the six to eight week level for vaginal delivery (see Fig. 15 above).

- Progress slowly.

- See Gym and the Pelvic Floor (page 91) for specific exercise guidelines when you return to the gym. Recent childbirth and pelvic surgery puts you in the 'at risk' category for returning to gym exercise.

Sex, Surgery and the Pelvic Floor

Sexual concerns can occur at any age but are more common post-birth, after pelvic surgery and with menopause. The cause can be physical, hormonal or psychological (or a mixture), so a combined treatment approach is often required.

Some women silently suffer sexual dysfunction because they are embarrassed to admit that their pelvic floor is so weak that they feel nothing. Their partner often comments that they feel less sensation during intercourse. Others avoid sex because of loss of urine or faeces during intercourse. (Researchers have identified that fluid loss with orgasm in some women can be from the prostatic-like glands that surround the female urethra.)[40]

A weakened pelvic floor can allow wind into the vagina during intercourse that causes an embarrassing farting noise. Some might have difficulty achieving an orgasm, or get pain during intercourse. Medication, major illness and depression can also lessen desire and vaginal lubrication.

Ten to 15% of women have pain with intercourse six months post-birth. This may be due to a dry vagina, perineal pain or excessive scarring from tears or episiotomy. Pain that persists this long after birth is not normal, and should be reviewed by an obstetrician and pelvic floor physiotherapist.[41]

Some women post-Caesarean have concerns about discomfort during sex from adhesions that cause the uterus to tip back, or due to a band of adhesions referring pain.[42]

While some women report improved health and normal sexual function after pelvic surgery, others report an adverse effect on their sexuality.

In one study, 38% of women reported overall dissatisfaction with sexual function after hysterectomy and prolapse surgery.[43] After hysterectomy, disruption of nerve supply leads to impaired lubrication and loss of sensation with orgasm. Bladder functioning can be affected along with defecation problems.[44]

A recent study shows that vaginal prolapse surgery results in more damage to nerves than abdominal prolapse surgery. Eighteen per cent of abdominally operated patients reported genital pain, whereas 37% of the vaginally operated group reported pain following surgery.[45] Surgeons are becoming more aware of performing nerve and blood vessel sparing pelvic surgery. The risks and benefits of any pelvic surgery should include accurate information on sexual dysfunction (decreased desire, orgasm, vaginal lubrication and pain). This needs to be routinely discussed when surgeons gain informed consent for gynaecological surgery.[46] Researchers and surgeons should be encouraged to look at which surgical approaches can preserve a woman's sexual functioning. With the increasing use of tape and mesh for reconstructive pelvic surgery, surgeons are reporting some unexpected side effects.

These include erosion of tapes, tape causing pressure damage to the nerve supplying the clitoris, and exposed mesh in the vagina.[47]

As part of addressing the high rate of 're-operations' for prolapse, women should know how to correctly activate and strengthen their pelvic floor muscles prior to surgery.

Learning correct muscle activation, and improving strength and endurance, will help provide support for the repair post operatively.

If a woman has an abnormal muscle pattern of bearing down on her pelvic floor when she tensions, then she will continue this same pattern postoperatively. This ongoing internal pressure down on the surgical repair may contribute to surgical failure.

Just as urodynamic studies are commonplace prior to pelvic surgery, the same priority should be placed on identifying the women who bear down incorrectly or have no active contraction. These at-risk women should be identified and retrained to reduce one factor that may contribute to surgical failure.

Important Tip

Before repair surgery or hysterectomy, women need strict guidelines about their return to activity post-operatively.

It is essential for women to receive verbal and written instruction about rest, bowel emptying, muscle activation, suitable activity, lifting, housework, sexual activity and return to work and sport. They need to plan for help at home during the recovery time.

Written guidelines are helpful so that partners know ahead of surgery what physical help is needed. This is important so that healing of the repair site is not compromised, as that may contribute to surgical failure. Repair takes place post-operatively as collagen is laid down to repair the surgical site. At 60 days post-operatively the wound should reach around 80% of its normal strength[48]. The remaining 20% of collagen may take from six months to two years to fully strengthen the surgical site.

If a woman returns to her normal duties and starts lifting more than two to three kilos before six weeks, she risks damage and breakdown of the surgical repair site. Return to normal duties and sport must be slow and graduated.

Smoking has been shown to slow healing post-operatively. Nicotine inhibits the formation of new blood vessels that are vital for healing and repair processes.

Pelvic floor physiotherapists are successfully treating post-operative pelvic pain. They use soft tissue mobilisation, myofascial release, muscle energy techniques, biofeedback, stabilising and strengthening exercises to treat adhesions related to chronic abdominal and pelvic pain and pelvic muscle spasms.

What are Kegel Exercises?

'Kegels' is a term used for pelvic floor exercises. This has caused confusion as some women think they may be a different type of exercise.

In 1948, Dr Arnold Kegel (who is credited with first teaching pelvic floor exercises) advised, 'It is a good idea in all cases that have been operated on for prolapse of the vagina vault or uterus, or in every postpartum woman to teach them how to contract the vaginal musculature and let them use this as a prophylactic measure.'[49]

Decreased vaginal sensation, muscle tone and orgasm improve with effective pelvic floor strengthening that focuses on building endurance and strength, particularly in the pubococcygeus muscle.

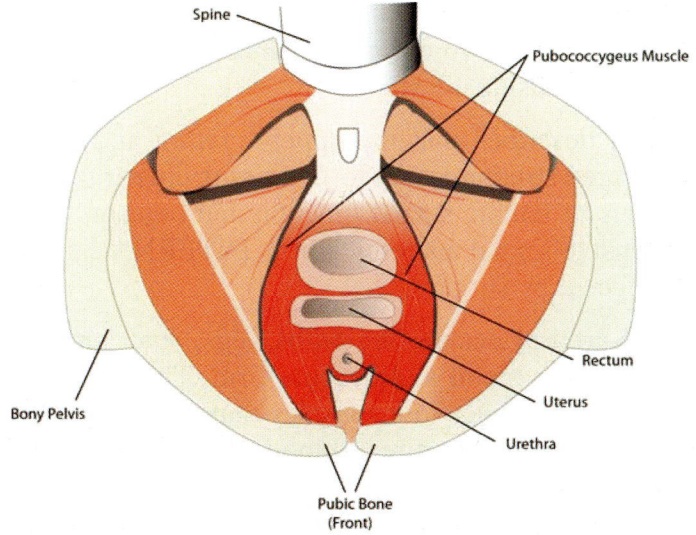

Fig. 16 – The Pelvic Floor from above

Dr Kegel applied the SSS theory to the Pubococcygeus muscle.[50]

SUPPORTIVE (for our internal organs)

SPHINCTERIC (closes the bladder and bowel sphincters)

SEXUAL (keeps vaginal walls firm and contracts with orgasm)

It's important to learn about your sexual anatomy to help you understand how the intensity of your orgasm is related to your pelvic floor muscle strength.

Female Sexual Anatomy

Most anatomy texts display external female genitalia and internal organs while totally leaving out the internal sexual anatomy. The clitoris is typically shown externally as a pea-sized bump. Dr Helen O'Connell, an Australian urologist, described how this 'bump' or glans is attached to a shaft about two to four centimetres long. Attached to the shaft are two clitoral legs about nine to 11 centimetres long that run back into the body in a wishbone type shape. Two clitoral bulbs of erectile tissue extend down to the area outside the vagina.

Dr O'Connell describes that the upper 'urethra and vagina are intimately related structures and form a tissue cluster that appears to be the locus of female sexual function and orgasm.'[51] Women have an extensive sexual anatomy that is INTERNAL and can be adversely affected by surgery.

When sexual arousal occurs, the bulbs, legs, shaft and glans of the clitoris fill with blood and become firm. The legs and bulbs are surrounded by pelvic floor muscles that contract to help the sensation of orgasm and direct blood flow to and from the clitoris.

With orgasm, contractions start in the smooth muscles of the fallopian tubes, uterus and glands surrounding the urethra, followed by contractions of voluntary muscles located in the pelvic floor, perineum and anal sphincter.[52] Along with other clitoral muscles, the pubococcygeus muscle contracts during orgasm and this forces blood out of erectile tissues to help create the potentially intense sensations of orgasm.

Weak, wasted muscles have fewer nerves and end plate receptors required to feel pleasurable sensations. Weak muscles have a poorer blood supply and cannot contract effectively to give the powerful sensations that usually occur with orgasm. Stronger muscles direct more blood flow to the clitoris and, combined with more powerful muscular contractions, the result is a more powerful orgasm.

Strong pelvic floor muscles = stronger orgasm.

Women with incontinence and prolapse have a significantly high rate of impaired sexuality.

Researchers looked at what happened to women's sexual function after they did pelvic floor exercises and improved their urinary incontinence. The women, who had vaginal pain, related a marked improvement - either less pain or complete relief of their pain. The women who experienced low sexual desire or difficulty gaining a climax reported improvement in their sexual function.[53] Pelvic floor physiotherapists are now at the front line of treating sexual dysfunction in women.[54]

The women who have a hyperactive (continually tight) pelvic floor will also have a decreased blood supply and sexual arousal disorders.[55] The constantly tight pelvic floor can cause pain on vaginal entry and during intercourse. Researchers have found that 61% of women with sexual pain disorders also complained of recurrent bacterial cystitis.[56]

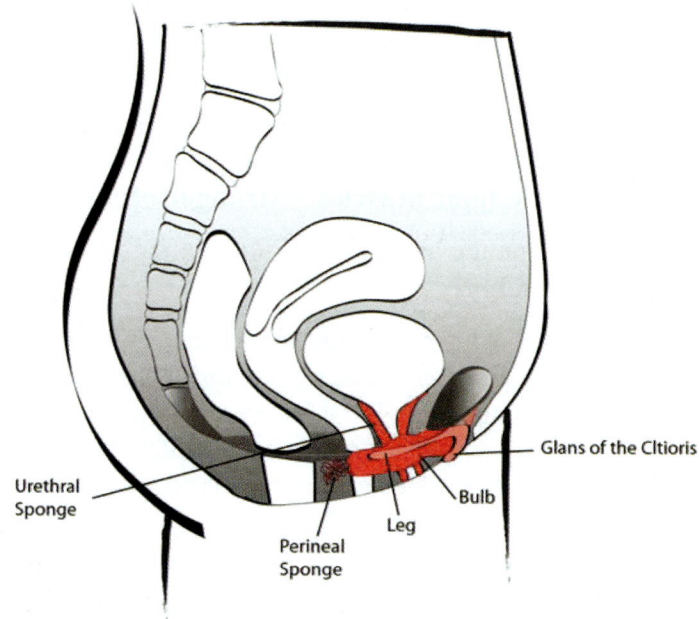

Fig. 17 - The Internal Parts of the Clitoris

88

Pain and the Pelvic Floor

If you experience pelvic floor pain, it can be due to:

- Scar tissue from one or more episiotomies causing vaginal pain

- Pelvic surgery

- The coccyx bone being broken during delivery or by falling onto the buttocks

- Pelvic organ prolapse and descending perineum

- Recto-anal ache that feels like a red-hot poker

- Interstitial cystitis (inflammation of the bladder lining)

- Endometriosis that is associated with painful periods and pain during intercourse (this pain can then progress on to chronic pelvic pain)

- Generalised vulvodynia

- Trigger points in the pelvis and buttocks.

Vulvodynia is a burning, throbbing or stinging sensation felt in the vulva, often along with pain and discomfort in the urethra or rectum. Vulval discomfort and pain is present with activity and in any position. The pain can limit a woman's ability to exercise or have intercourse.

Vulvodynia can be caused by pelvic or vulvovaginal surgery, childbirth, injury to hips or back (e.g. a herniated disc), a fall onto the buttocks, back surgery and spinal stenosis (narrowing of the canal around the spinal cord). Researchers in Boston showed that women who experienced pain when first using tampons were seven to eight times more likely to have vulval pain later in life.[57] If these women continue to have intercourse without arousal and in the presence of pain, their condition will worsen.

Intense vulval burning can be due to trauma or entrapment of the nerves supplying the pelvic floor. Treatment may include referral to an urologist, a dermatologist (for associated skin infections) and a physiotherapist for treatment of the spine and pelvic floor. Trigger points, pelvic floor muscle spasms, tight bands and scar tissue can be present in the pelvic floor as well as trigger points and tightness in buttock muscles.

Muscle spasms and trigger points develop in the pelvic floor when a sufferer walks around for months or years with continuous pelvic floor tension caused by pain and burning. When a muscle is excessively worked and overloaded, an area in the muscle can become hyper-irritable and result in pain, producing trigger points that can refer pain to other areas.[58]

Pelvic floor physiotherapy is directed towards muscle relaxation, shutting down the painful trigger points, soft tissue releases and correct muscle activation. Trigger points can be located in the pelvis, abdomen and buttocks as well as the pelvic floor. Fibromyalgia and irritable bowel syndrome are associated chronic pain syndromes that will contribute to the ongoing pain and stress of vulvodynia.

To learn more about vulvodynia, visit www.nva.org

Sexually Transmitted Disease

Burning when urinating, low abdominal pain and painful intercourse are also symptoms of sexually transmitted disease.

To learn more about STDs, visit
http://womenshealth.gov/faq/stdsgen.htm

Gym and the Pelvic Floor

While YOU know you cannot find or tension your pelvic floor muscles, or that you leak when you sneeze, or that your bladder gets urgent, your gym instructor has absolutely NO IDEA of your pelvic floor status. Not only does your gym instructor have no idea about your pelvic floor, they might also have little idea about how to prevent aggravating your present problems. They will guide you on all types of exercises without knowing about the special needs of your pelvic floor. The pelvic floor is one forgotten group of muscles that is rarely trained.

You must bring any pelvic floor problems to your gym's instructor's attention. If an instructor has their client's best interest in mind, they will refer you to a pelvic floor physiotherapist and modify your gym programme.

If you have a strong, problem-free pelvic floor, then starting a gym programme will strengthen all muscles in your body, including your pelvic floor.

Important Tip

Before starting a gym programme, all women should train their pelvic floor and deep abdominal area before adding weights.

Red flag questions are ones that let the trainer know if their client has any pelvic floor problems or if they are at risk of developing problems. How can any instructor be alerted to potential pelvic floor problems if they do not ask questions relevant to your pelvic floor function?

RED FLAG QUESTIONS that should be asked before commencing a gym programme are:

- Do you lose any urine when you cough, sneeze or run?

- Does your bladder become urgent?

- Did you have a difficult delivery?

- Have you had a Caesarean delivery?

- Did you experience any pain from pelvic instability during pregnancy?

- Do you have any separation of your tummy muscles?

- Post-birth, did your doctor find any prolapse?

- Have you had any pelvic or spinal surgery?

- Do you have any concerns with your bowel control?

- Are you unsure about how to contract your pelvic floor muscles correctly? (Not all women know how to do this correctly).

Answering 'yes' to one or more of these questions indicates a need to modify your gym activities and learn the correct pelvic floor and core muscle coordination. What happens at your waist when performing an exercise is the clue to your core control.

Ask your trainer to observe what happens at your abdomen as you exercise. If your waist draws back firmly and creases strongly, then you have learned to substitute outer abdominal muscles, instead of tensioning and holding pelvic floor and core muscles to perform the exercise.

Exercise Guidelines for Red Flag Clients

1. Avoid any curl-up abdominals and heavy weights

Prescribing sit-ups, curl-ups, medicine ball rotations, double leg lifts or Fitball crunches for abdominal strengthening of unfit, post-birth or menopausal women is the quickest way to help promote pelvic floor dysfunction. These abdominal exercises will forcefully push internal pressure down on your pelvic floor every time you curl up. Unless you have a strong pelvic floor that you can firmly tension to resist this downward pressure, then you are promoting internal straining. This damage presents as bladder urgency, increased leaking and maybe vaginal prolapse. I cannot stress strongly enough that these are unsuitable exercises for an 'at risk' pelvic floor.

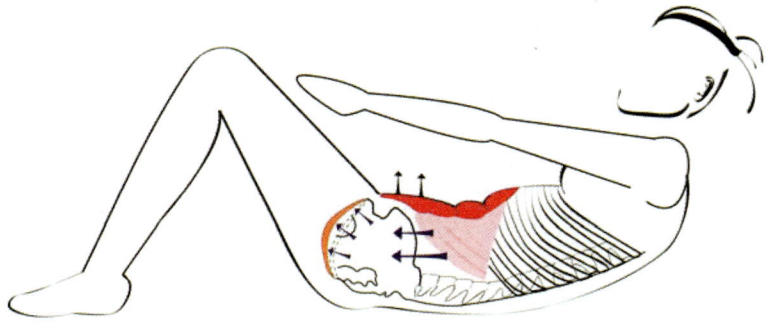

Repeated sit-ups can cause urgency, urge incontinence and prolapse.

Fig. 18 - Effect of Curl-ups on a Weak Pelvic Floor and Transversus

2. Focus on core strengthening exercises

Focus on correct posture during all exercises as this keeps your core muscles activated while you perform an exercise.

Suitable Exercises for RED FLAG Clients

- Pool-hydrotherapy

- Seated bike work

- Treadmill – keeping it flat initially

- Tai Chi

- Seated ball balancing with arm movement
- Light arm weights – military press, biceps, triceps, deltoid, upright row
- Lying and seated stretch band exercises
- Four-point kneel, opposite arm/leg holds
- Floor supine bridging holds
- Basic Pilates reformer exercises
- Pilates mat exercises
- Balance cushion activities
- Cool down with a stretching programme.

Spend four to six weeks working through this programme before adding progressions.

Progressions are made by:

- Increasing repetitions
- Increasing sets
- Increasing light weights
- Increasing band resistance
- Increasing cardio time on bike and walker.

Take four to six months to work through the above progressions.

When you perform an exercise, be aware of tensioning your pelvic floor prior to and during the exercise.

Progressions

- Standing stretch band exercises with arms and legs
- Standing on balance cushion with stretch band arm exercises

- Step-ups (start with lower step)

- Wall squats with fitball

- Regular squats (correct technique vital)

- Seated weight machines – lat pull down, seated row, leg press (lighter weights)

- Wall push-ups/bent knee prone push-ups

- Fitball under head (bridge position) with slow arm movements

- Prone walk out over Fitball with weight on hands (maintain neutral spine).

After three to four months on this programme, you will be more aware of your pelvic floor strength and exercise limitations.

NEVER perform an exercise that pushes your pelvic floor downwards and bulges your tummy forwards.

To exercise safely, you must be able to tension and hold your pelvic floor and lower tummy before and during the exercise.

Progress weights slowly and carefully.

Remember that a heavy upper body weight needs strong core strength before and during the lift.

Focus on maintaining correct posture when doing any exercise.

Important Tip

> **To avoid embarrassment for client or trainer, red flag questions can be included in a written questionnaire the client completes prior to beginning any programme.**

Menopause and the Pelvic Floor

It is likely that your pelvic floor will start to misbehave around the time of peri-menopause. Menopause officially happens when you have not had a period for 12 months. If you have ignored your pelvic floor up until now, then menopause is going to make you take notice. Milder symptoms that you previously accepted may become more marked.

What pelvic floor problems occur at menopause?

1. Leaking when you walk or exercise

Urine loss can worsen with menopause due to the drop in oestrogen levels. The lining of the urethra becomes softer and this reduces the closing pressure at the base of the bladder. This loss can be reversed by correctly tensioning and strengthening the pelvic floor muscles.

Maybe you have stopped exercising and put on weight. The extra pressure down on your pelvic floor can aggravate stress loss and urgency. You want to start exercising, but urine loss, perceived lack of time or poor self-esteem may stop you from even getting started.

Important Tip

> **Do not stop exercising if you leak. Continence guards inserted vaginally under the bladder neck can relieve urine loss while exercising.**

'If you don't use it, you will lose it'. This applies to muscle strength in all our muscles, particularly the pelvic floor.

Make a list of which activities you enjoy, and start with the easiest one.

In our clinic, clients attend hydrotherapy, Tai Chi, exercise classes with stretch bands, stationary bike riding or a walking programme, as their re-introduction to exercise.

Many shopping centres run free walking group sessions. Make a plan to do some exercise EVERY DAY of your life. If it seems too difficult to get started, get advice from a physiotherapist, exercise physiologist or trainer. Be sure they are aware of your pelvic floor issues.

Another reason to control weight gain at menopause is to avoid the fastest growing disease in the world – diabetes. Women who are both overweight and have Type II diabetes have a 50 to 70% increased risk of incontinence.[59] Post menopausal diabetic women are more likely to develop severe urinary incontinence[60] and increased risk of urinary tract infections.[61] A recent study of pre-diabetic, overweight women showed that the group who exercised and changed their diet reduced their stress incontinence and their risk of developing Type II diabetes.[62]

To learn more about diabetes, visit www.diabetes.com.au

2. Prolapse

What is prolapse?

Prolapse is a common condition that women don't discuss. It is caused by a pelvic organ (bladder, bowel or uterus) bulging down into the vagina because the vaginal fascial supports have been torn – due, for example, to childbirth, straining as a result of constipation, heavy lifting or coughing. The bladder and urethra can bulge down into the front vaginal wall; the bowel and intestine can bulge down into the back vaginal wall and the uterus can move down towards the vaginal opening.

What are the symptoms?

Prolapse may be present without any symptoms or it may cause an obvious bulge along with urinary, bowel and sexual dysfunction. Some women will have no other symptoms apart from an inner vaginal bulge, while others report lower backache, lower abdominal, vaginal or groin ache and heaviness that is worse at the end of the day. Other women first notice a prolapse when they feel a bulge at their vaginal opening.

Risk of prolapse

There is an increased risk of prolapse at menopause in women with several children and an increased waist measurement.[63] Smoking and heavy physical work increase the risk of prolapse. If your mother had a prolapse, then you have a three-fold increased risk of having prolapse.[64]

Dos and don'ts

If you have any or a combination of the above factors, then it's important to address the aggravating factors and strengthen your pelvic floor. When the muscles under your pelvic organs no longer give support, and the ligaments from above don't hold them up, then prolapse can occur when you continue to lift heavy objects or strain to empty your bowel. Some women develop prolapse after weeks of prolonged coughing due to a chest infection. Others notice that during and after a severe lower back injury, they have less control over their pelvic floor. Some relate prolapse after they slip down the stairs, after picking up their grandchildren or when they start a gym programme.

Non-surgical treatment of prolapse

A type of non-surgical treatment of prolapse, which is beneficial and cost effective, is the insertion of a vaginal pessary. Pessary supports are frequently used to reduce vaginal and uterine vault prolapse. Once the correct type and size of pessary has been fitted, it is then time to start an intensive pelvic floor muscle-strengthening programme, combined with vaginal oestrogen cream.

Doing strengthening exercises while the pessary is supporting the pelvic organs will improve the ability of the pelvic floor muscles to support these organs once the pessary is removed. As well as strength, your pelvic floor needs to provide support for long periods of time (endurance). When you walk or stand during the day, your pelvic floor needs endurance to stay switched on in a supporting mode. If it lacks strength and endurance then a prolapse will bulge more towards the end of the day.

A pessary should be removed, left out overnight and then reinserted as often as needed. It can be used during pregnancy and for relief of urinary incontinence as well as prolapse. If a woman is unable to remove the pessary by herself, then the pessary needs to be reviewed by her Doctor every three months for removal, inspection of vaginal walls, cleaning and reinsertion. Women who have had a hysterectomy, who have a shortened vaginal length, a higher number of children and an open vagina will often fail to retain a pessary.[65]

Surgery for prolapse

Women who have undergone surgical repair of their prolapse can expect that 30% of initial repairs and 50% of second surgical repairs will fail. Studies show that after one year, successful pessary treatment can be as effective as surgery. A long-term follow-up study is underway to determine if the results can be sustained.[66]

The risk of prolapse is increased by:

- Repeated heavy lifting
- Straining to empty your bowel
- Sit-ups, curl-ups or double leg lifts
- Not strengthening after childbirth or pelvic surgery
- Prolonged bouts of coughing

- Increasing abdominal fat
- Slumping when you sit or stand
- Avoiding daily pelvic floor exercises.

Reduce the risk of prolapse by:

- Weight loss
- Pelvic floor strength exercises
- Orgasm
- Avoiding heavy lifting
- Easy bowel opening
- An upright spinal posture
- Giving up smoking, which causes coughing
- Controlling allergies, which aggravate sneezing.

3. Bladder Urgency

With urgency, you empty your bladder more often to avoid accidents. You learn the location of every toilet before going on a shopping trip. You avoid long trips on public transport. When you turn on a tap, put a key in the door or head to the toilet, your bladder refuses to hold on and gets a mind of its own. When you get out of bed in the morning, your urgent bladder makes you curse as it leaks on the way to the bathroom – not the best way to start your day.

Urgency may indicate that the muscle that tensions the sphincters around the urethra and the base of the bladder is not working. This muscle is your body's inbuilt system to control your urgency.

Don't be fooled by thinking that tightening your anal sphincter is the correct exercise. When you can gently tension up the urethra at the front of your pelvic floor, you will start to control urgency and urine loss. After learning the correct tensioning, always progress with exercises to improve endurance and strength.

Important Tip

> **Bladder urgency after exercise or heavy work is a warning sign.**

Does your bladder get urgent after exercise or heavy gardening? This urgency is telling you that your level of exercise is too difficult as it is causing too much pressure down on your bladder. Your pelvic floor is not yet strong enough to counter that downward pressure. Keep strengthening your pelvic floor and ask for easier exercise options.

4. Urinary Tract Infections

Hormonal changes with the cessation of menstruation cause lower oestrogen, progesterone and testosterone levels. You may experience more urinary tract infections (UTIs) as the urethral and vaginal tissues start to thin.

You may notice decreased vaginal secretions during intercourse. This can aggravate UTIs and make intercourse unpleasant. Some women benefit from using a vaginal oestrogen cream or tablet.

A personal lubricant will help reduce discomfort during intercourse and prevent urethral irritation.

A natural product without chemical preservatives or parabens is SYLK. It is available in pharmacies and supermarkets in Australia and New Zealand. Visit www.sylk.com.au for more information.

Many women relate improvement of UTIs and bladder emptying after they strengthen their pelvic floor.

Habits to prevent UTIs

- Avoid caffeine and drink more water. Urinary alkalisers help to relieve burning symptoms.

- Avoid artificial sweeteners as they can cause urgency. Some diet soft drinks contain a double bladder whammy of caffeine and artificial sweeteners.

- Take cranberry tablets regularly. Cranberry helps to prevent the e-coli bacteria from attaching to your urethral and bladder walls and triggering a UTI. Eighty-five per cent of infections are caused by these bacteria.[67]

- Avoid douches and vaginal sprays that may irritate the urethra. Look for any chemicals listed on the container that have the potential to irritate your urethra.

- Before and after intercourse, wash your pelvic area to reduce bacteria. After intercourse, empty your bladder and take a cranberry tablet. Avoid intercourse positions that focus on thrusting towards your front vaginal wall, and use a vaginal lubricant. (Your urethra lies on your front vaginal wall).

- After emptying your bowel, always wipe from front to back. Either wash your anal area or carry a pack of wipes. This is to prevent the e-coli bacteria from migrating forward to your urethral entrance. The strings of your tampon can pick up the e-coli bacteria and transfer them forwards.

- Strengthen your pelvic floor muscles. Improving the muscular support under your bladder can help it to empty more fully. A bladder that does not fully empty is more prone to UTIs.

Most women who develop a UTI require antibiotics QUICKLY to settle the symptoms.

Do you continue to experience frequency, burning and pain above your pubic bone even when your mid-stream urine is free of bacteria when tested?

This could be due to interstitial cystitis (IC) or painful bladder syndrome, and will need investigation by an urologist. A recent study reports that only 9.4% of women with IC who get urinary infection type pain have a positive urine culture. The painful flare-ups are usually not associated with UTI's and are likely to be due to triggering of other painful mechanisms associated with IC[68]. Painful trigger points causing the UTI type pain are often found in these women, who usually gain relief after treatment of those trigger points. For more information, visit www.ichelp.org

5. Changes to your Sex Drive

A lower sex drive can be related to relationship difficulties, tiredness from trying to juggle work while caring for challenging teenagers or aging parents, or a work stressed partner. Add to that mix your own feelings about your changing body shape. Your body is telling you to start thinking about your own life, feelings and aspirations, and to spend some time improving your quality of life instead of doing this for everyone else.

Your sex drive is not meant to just go away. Your fertility will decline, but it is normal for sexual desire to continue in women until old age. Research suggests that, with aging and natural menopause, it's normal for a gradual decline in sexual interest and response.

Other research indicates that the less attractive a woman thinks she is, the more likely she is to report a decline in sexual desire. Women who lose their sexual desire as they age might be reacting to their own body image rather than to hormonal changes.[69] A lower sex drive at menopause has been related to lower levels of oestrogen, androgens and testosterone.[70] New studies on HRT show that it can make incontinence worse in affected women and cause urinary incontinence in previously unaffected women.[71]

Researchers think it is too simplistic to 'medicalise menopause' and try to find a 'cure' for loss of sexual desire with hormone replacement.

Women are concerned with their weight and about how their body looks and functions. Their sexuality can be affected by loss of economic, social and political control in their lives. If a woman is criticised or abused in her relationships; if she does not trust her partner; if she has ongoing pain; is depressed, fearful or feels that her life has no meaning, then these feelings are likely to be reflected in her sexual response.

Many women do not feel distressed by their lack of interest in, or response to sex. So, if a woman does not feel distressed about lack of response, is it a problem?[72]

Try observing the women who have an easier passage through menopause. They have satisfying relationships, exercise regularly, eat lots of fresh food, get enough sleep, have a network of friends, pursue their own interests and activities and have learned to control their stress reaction. They give themselves permission to take time out. They don't live their lives through their grown-up children, but focus on their own work and dreams.

The Wisdom of Menopause by Dr. Christiane Northrup contains a wealth of knowledge to help guide you through this transitional life stage. Visit her website at www.drnorthrup.com

The Older Pelvic Floor

Age is NO barrier to learning pelvic floor exercises.

Women in their 70s and 80s regularly learn to locate and strengthen their pelvic floor muscles, and improve bladder control. Their pelvic floor and spine will also benefit from learning better postural control. A recent study shows that pelvic floor muscles work more effectively when a woman sits upright, so avoid slumping your lower back. Sit tall and teach your pelvic floor muscles to stay switched on, supporting your pelvic organs as well as your spine.

Conditions such as diabetes, Parkinson's, muscular sclerosis, spinal cord injury, dementia and stroke can affect brain signals to your bladder and bowel, and lessen control. These conditions can severely limit mobility and the ability to care for yourself. Excess weight, high caffeine intake and smoking are factors that aggravate incontinence in older age. Lack of exercise leads to muscle wasting, loss of balance and incontinence.

Older women take more drugs and this has been shown to cause higher rates of urinary incontinence.[73]

Ask your doctor and pharmacist to review your medication so you know which drugs cause bladder incontinence or slow down your bowel, causing constipation. A back-up of stools will cause urinary incontinence.

Vaginal dryness and muscle wasting that causes incontinence can be helped with oestrogen cream.

Urge incontinence is more common in older women, and again pelvic floor exercises are the first line of defence. Our bodies have a built-in system that relaxes the urgent bladder when the pelvic floor muscles are contracted.

As women age, about 50% develop night-time frequency (nocturia). An urgent bladder forces you to get up from two to six times a night to empty your bladder. This can affect your health and cause ongoing tiredness during the day. This tiredness may lead to a fall and the risk of a broken bone. Nocturia is aggravated by some heart and kidney problems, incomplete bladder emptying, some medications (sedatives, diuretics), too much alcohol, caffeine and artificial sweeteners. Sleep apnoea and diabetes may also aggravate this night-time frequency.

Treatment can include a review of your medications, reducing caffeine and alcohol, eliminating artificial sweeteners, wearing compression stockings to control swollen ankles, an afternoon rest, testing your urine for infection and other specialised tests. A stronger pelvic floor will stop urine loss as you walk to the toilet at night.

Arthritis and immobility make it difficult for some frail, elderly or disabled people to reach the toilet in time. To help maintain their continence and independence it is vital to look at toilet placement, easy access, safe rails for support and removing obstacles that could cause a fall.

□ **Case Study** □

Jeanie, aged 72, was referred by her doctor due to strong bladder pain before she urinated, stress incontinence and strong bearing down to open her bowel. Jeanie's husband had died 18 months earlier and her ongoing stress was obvious in her tense body posture. Jeanie sat slumped with her shoulders hunched and her waist drawn back tightly. She demonstrated using this same posture when she passed urine and opened her bowel.

Jeanie was shown how to control her sitting and standing posture. She added more dietary fibre and fresh food to her diet and learned how to sit and release her abdominal tension when using her bladder and bowel.

At her second visit, she excitedly related that her bladder pain was minimal and her bowel opened every day without straining. Her bladder had not leaked (and she had not yet been instructed in pelvic floor activation). She learned to locate her pelvic floor and to be aware of her gentle pelvic floor tensioning, initially in side lying – gentle, because she had never consciously used or strengthened her pelvic floor. Over the next month, she then progressed this tensioning to sitting and standing.

Jeannie's quality of life improved markedly once she had less pain and fear. As a result of her correct pelvic floor patterns, she is now regaining full bladder control in all aspects of her life.

Pelvic Floor Therapy to Treat Incontinence

In Australia, the government recognises that physiotherapy is a highly effective, cost saving treatment for incontinence.

Costs: physiotherapy vs surgery

Physiotherapy treatment of incontinence (when another medical condition such as arthritis or back pain is also present) is available through Medicare. To access treatment through the Medicare Extended Primary Care plan, a referral from your GP is required. This treatment was made available because Australian studies show the effectiveness of pelvic floor physiotherapy in curing or improving incontinence. The cost of the average episode with a physiotherapist is around $300 to $400 compared to an estimated $4,000 to $6,000 for colposuspension surgery.[74]

Physiotherapy treatment may include biofeedback and muscle stimulation using a vaginal or anal electrode.

The biofeedback electrode uses visual or auditory signals to encourage pelvic floor muscle tensioning. It can also be used to learn how to relax overly tight muscles.

Connecting the electrode to a muscle stimulator allows electrical currents to activate weak muscles or to calm down an overactive bladder. Once pelvic floor muscle activation is learned, Physiotherapists introduce strength exercises to progress voluntary control.

Osteoporosis

Many women are unaware of this common, disabling disease process in their bodies. The largest amount of bone loss occurs in the five years post-menopause.

Osteoporosis Australia reports that one in two women and one in three men over 60 will have a fracture from osteoporosis.

Bone mass is greatest in the early 20s, so it's essential that children and teenagers build their bone density with regular exercise and a calcium rich diet. It's too late to build sufficient bone density in your late 20s and 30s. Teenagers who regularly consume carbonated drinks, eat a nutrient poor diet and avoid regular physical activity, increase their risk of developing osteoporosis. The phosphates in soft drinks affect the absorption of calcium. Young women, who regularly drink more than the daily recommended level of alcohol and also smoke, increase their risk of osteoporosis. Women and girls who severely restrict their food intake to stay thin share the same risk.

Young female athletes are prone to osteoporosis, when their heavy training schedule, combined with calorie controlled eating, causes their periods to stop or become irregular. This lowers their normal hormonal levels and their bodies take calcium from existing bones. Gymnasts, swimmers, rowers and dancers are in the high risk groups.

At risk athletes and pre- and post-menopausal women can check their bone density levels with a DEXA scan. A referral for this scan may be obtained through your GP.

Visit www.osteoporosis.org.au to learn more.

The three most important factors that affect bone growth are:

- Nutrition (adequate daily intake of calcium rich foods)
- Hormonal activity (oestrogen and progesterone play a role in bone growth)

- Exercise (progressive strength exercises and weight-bearing aerobic activity).

Exercise needs to be tailored to the individual, depending on the presence or stage of the disease.

A pre-menopausal woman can benefit from a continued weights programme, dancing and tennis. However, an older woman diagnosed with an osteoporotic vertebral fracture will need a carefully guided programme, often starting with hydrotherapy once her pain has settled. A graduated exercise programme should focus on strengthening spinal extensor muscles, as this has been shown to be most effective in preventing further spinal fractures. Exercises that involve spinal bending and twisting should be avoided.[75]

Balance, postural control and strength exercises are vital to prevent falls, which can cause further fractures. Specific balance and strength classes as well as Tai Chi will improve balance and lessen the risk of falling in elderly people.

What does osteoporosis have to do with the pelvic floor?

If osteoporosis progresses, height is lost as the vertebrae compress and the posture becomes stooped. The abdomen will bulge forwards. This in turn puts more pressure down on the bladder and bowel, causing urgency and incontinence.

Pelvic floor exercises will be more effective if they are learned earlier in life rather than waiting until problems begin.

The Pelvic Floor for Life

Typically, we pass through childhood into adolescence and adult years and don't give our pelvic floor a second thought until pregnancy and birthing. Then our pelvic 'flaw' becomes all too evident. To change the near epidemic level of pelvic floor problems currently being experienced by women, start to put the information you have read into action today.

- Why wait until you are pregnant?

- Why wait until you experience sexual dysfunction?

- Why wait until you cannot control your bladder or bowel?

- Why wait until you are menopausal?

- Why wait until a prolapse suddenly presents?

Starting a new set of daily habits will help protect and benefit your pelvic floor.

- Control your posture to keep your core muscles active

- Use the new position to empty your bowel. Keep your bowel contents soft

- Persist until you learn the correct pelvic floor tensioning then continue to strengthen and use your pelvic floor muscles every day of your life

- Stop lifting weights that are too heavy for your body

- Keep exercising regularly and control your weight. Choose exercises that target your core muscles and avoid damaging abdominal work

- After childbirth, abdominal, pelvic or spinal surgery, rehab your core muscles for five to six months. Consult a pelvic floor physio to guide your progress.

Take control of your pelvic floor. It is never too late to improve problems by adopting new habits and strengthening your muscles. Don't accept worsening problems as part of being female. You are now aware of how much can be done to correct and prevent problems. If you talk to other women about the information contained in this book, you will be amazed how this gives them the cue to talk about their own problems.

Become a part of passing on the correct knowledge about treatment and prevention of pelvic floor problems. Talk to your daughters when they are small and want to listen; counsel young athletes about damaging exercise routines; give this book to young mums; share this information with women who no longer enjoy sex and talk to your friends whose lives are controlled by trips to the toilet.

I hope that this information helps you make informed decisions about your pelvic floor. Never, ever give up on your pelvic floor.

My final words are to urge you to include this information in your female wisdom to be passed on from generation to generation of women.

Resources

To find a Pelvic Floor Physiotherapist

- Call the Australian Physiotherapy Association in your state.

- Ask your local physiotherapist, doctor, community health nurse, gynaecologist or pharmacist for the name of a local pelvic floor physiotherapist.

- Call the Continence Foundation as they have a list of pelvic floor physiotherapists.

Websites

Physiotherapy Associations

Australian Physiotherapy Association www.physiotherapy.asn.au

Ph: 03 9543 9199

New Zealand Physiotherapy Assoc. www.physiotherapy.org.nz

Ph: 64 4 801 6500

Singapore Physiotherapy Assoc. www.physiotherapy.org.sg

U.K. Physiotherapy Association www.csp.org.uk

Ph: 020 7306 6666

U.S.A. Physical Therapy Assoc. www.apta.org

Ph: 800/999-2782

Canadian Physiotherapy Assoc. www.physiotherapy.ca

Ph: 1 800 387 8679

Irish Society of Charted Physio. www.iscp.ie

Ph: 00353(0)1 4022148

Netherlands Physiotherapy Assoc. www.kngf.nl

Ph: +31 3346 72 900

European Physiotherapy Associations www.cebp.nl/?NODE=85

Continence Organisations

Australian Continence Foundation www.continence.org.au

Ph: 1800 33 00 66

N.Z. Continence Association www.continence.org.nz

Ph: 0800 650 659

Singapore Continence Association
www.sfcs.org.sg/sfc_links.htm

Ph: 65-6787 0337

U.K. Continence Foundation www.continence-foundation.org.uk

Ph: 0845 345 0165

U.S.A. Continence Association www.nafc.org

Ph: 1 800 BLADDER (252 3337)

Canadian Continence Association www.continence-fdn.ca

Ph: 705 750-4600

Irish Continence Society www.continence.ie

Netherlands Continence Association. www.pelvicfloor.nl

Ph: 31 2069 70 304

Worldwide Continence Organization
www.continenceworldwide.org/contorg.html

Glossary of Terms

Colposuspension surgery	Operation to correct stress incontinence. It lifts the uterus and bladder back up. Colposuspension comes from the Greek name for the vagina - colpos
c-section	Caesarean section birth
DEXA	Dual Energy X-ray Absorptiometry, or DEXA scanning, is currently the most widely used method to measure bone mineral density
Episiotomy	Surgical incision of the perineum during childbirth to facilitate delivery
Fascia	The tough, thin, translucent membrane (similar to what you pull off meat) that joins the sections of a muscle
Pelvic instability	A condition causing pain and varying degrees of mobility in joints of the pelvis
Pubic symphysis	The midline cartilaginous joint that unites the left and right pubic bones
Rectus diastasis	Separation of the rectus abdominis muscle which occurs during pregnancy
Relaxin	A hormone produced during pregnancy that softens pelvic joints in preparation for delivery
Sacroiliac joint pain	Pain in the joints that lie next to the base of the spine and connect the sacrum with the pelvis
Sciatic pain	Pain in the buttock or leg due to irritation of the sciatic nerve
Urodynamics studies	Tests done on the bladder to reproduce symptoms so the problem can be treated
UTI	Urinary tract infection
Vulvodynia	Burning, throbbing or stinging sensation felt in the vulva, often along with pain and discomfort in the urethra or rectum

References

[1] Hagen et al. 2004 Conservative management of pelvic organ prolapse in women. The Cochrane Database of Systematic Reviews, http://www.cochrane.org/reviews/en/ab003882.html

[2] Bai SW, Jeon MJ, Kim JY, Chung KA, Kim SK, and Park KH. 2002 Relationship between stress urinary incontinence and pelvic organ prolapse. Int Urogyn J.13(4):256-260.

[3] De Lancey J. 2005. The hidden epidemic of pelvic floor dysfunction. J.American Journal of Ob. & Gyn. 192(5),1488-1495.

[4] Thompson JA, and O'Sullivan PB, Briffa NK, Neumann P. 2006 Differences in muscle activation patterns during pelvic floor muscle contraction and valsalva manouevre. Neurourol Urodyn 25(2)148-155.

[5] Meyer S, Hohlfeld P, Achtari C, Russolo A. and de Grandi P. 2000. Birth trauma: short and long term effects of forceps delivery compared with spontaneous delivery on various pelvic floor parameters. BJOG Vol.107(11):1360-1370.

[6] Sapsford R. Richardson C. and Stanton WR. 2006 Sitting posture affects pelvic floor activity in parous women: An observational study. Aust J Physio 52(3):219-222

[7] Kiff ES, Barnes PR, Swash M. 1984 Evidence of pudendal neuropathy in patients with perineal descent and chronic straining at stool. Gut 25:1279-1282.

[8] Hodges PW 2006. Low back pain and the pelvic floor. In: The Pelvic Floor, Carriere B. & Markel-Zeldt C (Eds), Thieme, Stuttgart.

[9] Thompson JA, and O'Sullivan PB. 2003 Levator plate movement during voluntary pelvic floor muscle contraction in subjects with incontinence and prolapse - a cross sectional study and review. Int Urogyn J Vol 14(2):84-88.

[10] Sapsford R. Hodges P. and Richardson C. 1997 Activation of the abdominal muscles is a normal response to contraction of the pelvic floor muscles. Conference abstract. International Continence Society, Yokohama, p117.

[11] Markwell S. 1998. Functional disorders of the anorectum and pain syndromes. In: Women's Health: A textbook for physiotherapists, Sapsford R. Bullock-Saxton J. and Markwell S. (Eds) WB Saunders Co. London p.357.

[12] Jorgsen S, Hein HO and Gyntelberg F. 1994 Heavy lifting at work and risk of genital prolapse and herniated lumbar disc in assistant nurses. Occup Med 44:47-49.

[13] Woodman PJ, Swift SE, O'Boyle AL, Valley MT, Bland DR, Kahn MA and Schaffer JI. 2006. Prevalence of severe pelvic organ prolapse in relation to job description and socioeconomic status: a multicentre cross-sectional study. Int Urogyn J. 17(4):340-345

[14] Haylen B.T. 2006 The retroverted prolapse: ignored to date but core to prolapse. Inter Urogyn J. 17(6):555-558.

[15] Subak LL, Johnson C, Johnson C, Whitcomb E, Boban D, Saxton J. and Brown JS, 2002, Does weight loss improve incontinence in moderately obese women? Inter Urogyn J.(2002) 13(1):40-43.

[16] Bernstein IT.1997. The pelvic floor muscles: Muscle thickness in healthy and urinary-incontinent women measured by perineal ultrasonography with reference to the effect of pelvic floor training. Estrogen receptor studies. Neurourol Urodyn 16(4):237-75.

[17] Minassian VA, Lovatsis D, Pascali D, Alarab M and Drutz HP. 2006. Effect of childhood dysfunctional voiding on urinary incontinence in adult women. O&G 107(6):1247-1251.

[18] Von Gontard A, Laufersweiler-Plass C. Backes M. Zerres K and Rudnik-Shoneborn S. 2001. Enuresis and urinary incontinence in children and adolescents with spinal muscular dystrophy. BJU Int .88(4)409-413.

[19] Alnaif B.& Drutz HP. 2001 The prevalence of urinary and fecal incontinence in Canadian secondary school teenage girls: questionnaire study and review of the literature. Int Urogyn J. 12(2):134-137.

[20] Nygaard IE, Thompson FL, Svengalis SL and Albright JP. 1994 Urinary incontinence in elite nulliparous athletes. Obstet Gynecol 84:183-187).

[21] Thyssen HH, Clevin L, Olesen S, Lose G. 2002. Urinary incontinence inn elite female athletes and dancers. Int Urogyn J. 13(1):15-17

[22] Bo K. Borgen JS. 2001 Prevalence of stress and urge urinary incontinence in elite athletes and controls. Med Sci Sports Ex. 33(11):1797-1802.

[23] Sampselle CM, Miller JM, Mims BL, DeLancey JO, Ashton-Miller and Antonakos CL. 1998. Effect of pelvic muscle exercise on transient incontinence during pregnancy and after birth. O&G. 91(3):406-412

[24] Eason E. Labrecque M. Marcoux S. and Mondor M. 2004. Effects of carrying a pregnancy and of method of delivery on urinary incontinence: a prospective cohort study. *BMC Pregnancy and Childbirth* 2004, 4:4.

[25] Bo K, Hagen LAHH, Voldner NV. 2006. Do pregnant women exercise their pelvic floor muscles? Int Urogyn J. 17(Supp 2):S175.

[26] Pool-Goudzwaard AL, Slieker ten Hove CPH, Vierhout ME, Mulder PH, Pool JJM, Snijdres CJ, Stoeckart R. Relations between pregnancy related low back pain, pelvic floor activity and pelvic floor dysfunction. Int Urogyn J (2005) 16: 468-474.

[27] Fynes M. 2003 Effect of pregnancy & delivery on post vaginal compartment. Proceedings, Int Continence Society 33rd Annual Meeting Florence.

[28] Elneil S. 2007 Vesico-Vaginal & Recto-Vaginal fistula in the developing world. ICS News, Issue no 5 January 2007, International Continence Society.

[29] Press J, Klein MC and von Dadelszen P. 2006. Mode of delivery and pelvic floor dysfunction: A systematic review of the literature on urinary and faecal incontinence and sexual dysfunction by mode of delivery. MedGenMed eJournal: http://www.medscape.com/viewarticle/521510

[30] De Tayrac R, Panel L, Masson G. and Mares P. 2006. Episiotomy and prevention of perineal and pelvic floor injuries. J Gyn Obst Biol Reprod (Paris) 2006 Feb;35(1 Suppl):1S24-1S31).

[31] Signorello LB, Harlow BL, Chekos, AK and Repke JT. 2001. Post partum sexual functioning and its relationship to perineal trauma: a retrospective cohort study of primiparous women. Am J Obstet Gynecol.184(5):881-8

[32] Dietz HP, Hyland G and Hay-Smith J. 2006. The assessment of levator trauma: A comparison between palpation and 4D pelvic floor ultrasound Neurourol Urodyn 25(5):424-427.

[33] Jack GS, Kikolova G, Vilain E, Raz S, Rodriguez L. 2006 Familial transmission of genitovaginal prolapse. .Int Urogyn J. 17(5):498-501.

[34] Sakala C. 2006 Comparing harms of vaginal and Caesarian birth: Maternity Centre Association's Systematic Review and Education and Quality Improvement Campaign. Childbirth Connection http://www.childbirthconnection.org/article.asp?ck=10271&ClickedLink=200 &area=2

[35] Groom KM, Paterson-Brown S. 2000. Third degree anal sphincter tears: are they clinically underdiagnosed? Gast. Int. 13(2):76-77.

[36] Eason E. Labrecque M. Marcoux S. and Mondor M. 2002. Anal incontinence after childbirth. CMAJ.2002 February 5;166(3):326-330.

[37] Chiarelli P. Murphy B. Cockburn J. 2003. Faecal incontinence after high risk delivery. Obstetrics and Gynecology 102(6):1299-1305.

[38] Chiarelli P, Murphy B and Cockburn J. 2004. Promoting urinary continence in postpartum women: 12 month follow-up data from a randomised controlled trial. Int. Urogyn. J.15(2):99-105.

[39] Spitznagle TM, Leong FC and Van Dillen LR. 2007. Prevalence of diastasis recti abdominis in a urogynecological patient population. Int Urogynl J. 18(3):321-328.

[40] Chalker R. 2000. The Clitoral Truth, Seven Stories Press, New York.

[41] Sneddon A, Ellwood D. Post Partum Care. Australian Doctor, April 30, 2004: p40

[42] Maternity Centre Association. 2006. "What every pregnant women needs to know about caesarian section." Childbirth Connection.

[43] Rogers R. Report from the 24th annual meeting of AUGS. Med Gen Med e-Journal, http://www.medscape.com/viewarticle/461719_6

[44] Trimbos JB, Maas CP, Deruiter MC, Peters AAW, Kenter GG. 2001. A nerve-sparing radical hysterectomy: Guidelines and feasibility in western patients. Int J Gynecol Cancer 11(3):180-186

[45] Roovers JPWR, Raart CH van der. 2006. Damage to vaginal innervation is more extensive during vaginal prolapse surgery than during abdominal prolapse surgery.Int Urogyn J. 17(Sup 2):S74

[46] Dragisic K, Milad M 2004 Sexual functioning and patient expectations of sexual functioning after hysterectomy. AJOG 190(5);1418-8.

[47] Brubaker L. 2006. Editorial: partner dyspareunia (hispareunia). Int. Urogyn. J. 17(4):311.

[48] Maxwell D. 2004. Surgical Techniques in Obstetrics and Gynaecology. Churchill Livingstone, New York.

[49] Kegel AH, 1948, The non surgical treatment of genital relaxation, West, Med & Surg. 31:213-216.

[50] Kegel AH, 1952, Sexual function of the P.C. muscle. Western J of Surgery,.Obst & Gyn 60;521-524.

[51] O'Connell HE, Sanjeevan KV, Hitson JM. 2005. Anatomy of the clitoris. J Urol. Oct;174(4 Pt 1):1189-95

[52] Selzer M Clarke S. Cohen L. Duncan P. Gage F. (Eds) 2006 Textbook of Neural Repair and Rehabilitation: Medical Neurorehabilitation. Cambridge University Press, London

[53] Beji NK, Yalcin O, Erkan HA. 2003. The effect of pelvic floor training on sexual function of treated patients. Int Urogyn J. 14(4):234-238

[54] Rosenbaum TY. 2006. The role of physiotherapy in sexual health: Is it evidenced based? J Chartered Physio in Women's Health. 99:1-5

[55] Graziottin A. 2004. Sexual pain disorders: Clinical approach. Urodinamica 14:105-111

[56] Salonia A, Zanni G, Nappi RE, Briganti A, Deho F, Fabbri F, Colombo R, Guazzoni G, Di Girolamo V, Rigatti P, Montorsi F. 2004. Sexual dysfunction is common in women with lower urinary tract symptoms and urinary incontinence: results of a cross sectional study. Eur Urol. 45(5):642-8.

[57] Harlow B. and Gunther-Stewart E. 2003. A population-based assessment of chronic unexplained vulvar pain: have we underestimated the prevalence of vulvodynia? JAMWA. 58(2):82-88.

[58] Travell J. & Simons D. 1983. Myofascial pain and Dysfunction: The trigger point manual. Williams &Wilkins, Baltimore MD

[59] Smith DB, A continence care approach for long term care facilities. Geriatric Nursing. Vol 19, Issue 2.81-86

[60] Jackson SL, Boyko EJ. And Fihn SD. 2005. Urinary incontinence and diabetes in postmenopausal women. Diab. Care 28(7):17301738.

[61] Smith DB. 2006. Urinary incontinence and diabetes: a review. J.Wound Ostomy & Cont. Nurs. 33(6):619-23.

[62] Knowler WC, Barrett-Connor E, Fowler SE, Hamman RF, Lachin JM, Walker EA and Nathan DM. 2002. Reduction in the incidence of type-2 diabetes with lifestyle intervention or Metformin. New Eng. J.Med. 346(6):393-403.

[63] How common is pelvic organ prolapse(and is this a normal finding)? Medscape Ob/Gyn&Womens Health Report from 24th annual meeting of AUGS http://www.medscape.com/viewarticle/461719_7

[64] Vierhout ME, Slieker ten Hove MC. 2006 Familial transmission of pelvic organ prolapse. 31st Ann Int Urogyn Assoc Meeting, Athens, Greece, Sept 6-9.

[65] Sheetle MS. and Jones P. 2006 Effect of vaginal pessaries on symptoms associated with pelvic organ prolapse. Obs & Gyn 108:93-99.

[66] Fernando RJ. Thakar R. Sultan AH. 2006. Are vaginal pessaries as effective as surgery in symptomatic pelvic organ prolapse? 31st Annual Int Urogyn. Assoc. Meeting, Athens, Greece, 6-9 Sept 2006.

[67] Avorn J, Monane M, Gurwitz JH, Glynn RJ, Choodnovskiy I, Lipsitz LA.et al.1994 Reduction of bacteriuria and pyuria after ingestion of cranberry juice. JAMA, 271(10);751-754.

[68] Stanford EJ and McMurphy C. 2006. There is a low incidence of bladder bacteriuria in painful bladder syndrome/interstitial cystitis patients followed longitudinally. Int Urogyn J. 17(Sup 2):S85

[69] Koch PB, Mansfield PK, Thurau D, Carey M. 2005. "Feeling Frumpy": the relationships between body image and sexual response changes in midlife women. J of Sex Res. 42(3):215-223.

[70] Northrup C. 2003. The Wisdom of Menopause. Bantam, New York

[71] Hunskaar S 2006 State-of-the-art address. Proceedings of I.C.S. 36th Annual Meeting. Christchurch.

[72] ARHP Clinical Proceedings - women's sexual health in midlife and beyond: introduction. From Medscape http://www.medscape.com/viewarticle/506390

[73] Nygaard IC, Thompson FL, Svengalis SL and Albright JP. 1996. Urinary incontinence in rural older women. J Am Ger Soc 44(9):1049-54.

[74] Neumann PB, Grimmer KA, Grant RE and Gill VA. 2005. Physiotherapy for female stress urinary incontinence: a multicentre observational study. Aust & N.Z. J of Ob & Gyn. 45(3):226-232

[75] MacKinnon JL (1988) Osteoporosis:a review. Physical Therapy 68:1533-1541).

[76] Smith MD, Coppieters MW and Hodges PW. 2007. Postural response of the pelvic floor and abdominal muscles in women with and without incontinence. Neuro Urodyn. 26(3):377-385.

Ordering

You can order *My Pelvic Flaw* in any of the following ways:

Online by visiting www.mypelvicfloor.com.au

Posting this form to: Redsok Publishing, P.O. Box 1881, Buderim, Qld 4556, Australia (Telephone +61 (0)7 5443 8005)

Faxing this form to +61 (0)7 5443 4349

NAME: _____

ADDRESS: _____

CITY: _____

POSTCODE: _____ COUNTRY: _____

DAYTIME PHONE: _____

EMAIL: _____

METHOD OF PAYMENT

CREDIT CARD (the charge slip will be mailed to you)

☐   Visa   ☐   MasterCard

Card number: _____

Expiration date: _____ / _____   ccv _____

Name on card: _____

Number of books ordered: _____

Price: $24.95 (Aust) each plus postage and handling

Thank you